# Perpetrators of Intimate Partner Sexual Violence

Research shows that intimate partner sexual violence (IPSV) is the most common form of sexual assault. Professional focus is often on the victim, but more information is needed about the perpetrators in order to have a fuller understanding of this crime. The very nature of IPSV – sexual assault within a relationship – means that professionals who work with victims must understand the dynamics of perpetrators as well.

This new book will distill the knowledge that exists about perpetrators of IPSV. It includes chapters by authors who have worked directly with IPSV perpetrators and covers important subjects such as addressing IPSV in batterer groups, police management strategies, the danger of IPSV to children, the different types of violence perpetrators use, and prevention approaches for young people. There is also still a widely held view that rapists are strangers in alleyways. This book is intended to educate professionals about who is a perpetrator, as well as to highlight the very real danger these perpetrators represent, including a heightened risk of lethality.

The contributors look at the social context of IPSV and the implications for prevention and provide hands-on knowledge to practitioners in a number of fields. The book may also be used within the academic context in fields such as social work, sociology, counseling, psychology, medicine, nursing, criminal justice, and law.

**Louise McOrmond–Plummer** is Research Associate at the West Virginia University Center on Violence, USA. She has twenty-five years of study, work and activism experience in the areas of domestic violence and sexual assault, with particular focus on intimate partner sexual violence.

**Jennifer Y. Levy-Peck**, PhD, is a clinical psychologist with more than thirty-five years of experience working with survivors of domestic violence and sexual assault, and has developed expertise in program development and victim advocacy. She is president of Levy-Peck Consulting, LLC.

**Patricia Easteal**, AM, is Professor of Law at the University of Canberra, Australia. She has twenty-plus years of research, writing, advocacy and teaching experience in the area of women and the law, domestic violence and sexual assault. She has written and/or edited 15 relevant books and more than 160 academic journal articles.

"*Perpetrators of Intimate Partner Sexual Violence* is an important and valuable contribution to our understanding of this widespread, yet understudied, form of violence. Noted scholars, practitioners and survivors offer new research as well as extensive intervention and prevention recommendations. This volume will prove most useful for all of us working to end sexual violence."

– *Kersti Yllo, Wheaton College, USA*

"The subjects of this comprehensive, well-researched, and disturbing collection are the men who have sexually assaulted a partner and the effects on the women and children who are victimized by them. The book is long overdue, much needed, and path-breaking."

– *Evan Stark, Rutgers University, USA*

"McOrmond-Plummer, Easteal and Levy-Peck have made a critical contribution to the field of violence against women with this multi-disciplinary book that addresses a highly understudied phenomena.

For far too long there has been a dearth of information about men who sexually abuse their intimate partners. This important book assembles leading experts from a variety of disciplines to address this void in an important way. For those who are working in the community with perpetrators, those working with women who have been victimized by their partners and others committed to ending violence against women, this book is essential reading.

This book contributes in an important way to furthering our understanding of IPSV as 'real rape' with very real consequences for society and most importantly, the lives of women who are victimized by their partners."

– *Raquel Bergen, Saint Joseph's University, USA*

# Perpetrators of Intimate Partner Sexual Violence

A multidisciplinary approach
to prevention, recognition, and
intervention

Edited by
Louise McOrmond-Plummer,
Jennifer Y. Levy-Peck
and Patricia Easteal

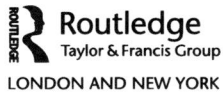
Routledge
Taylor & Francis Group

LONDON AND NEW YORK

First published 2017
by Routledge
2 Park Square, Milton Park, Abingdon, Oxon OX14 4RN

and by Routledge
711 Third Avenue, New York, NY 10017

Routledge is an imprint of the Taylor & Francis Group,
an informa business

*British Library Cataloguing in Publication Data*
A catalogue record for this book is available from the British Library

*Library of Congress Cataloging in Publication Data*
A catalog record for this book has been requested

ISBN: 978-1-138-91044-7 (hbk)
ISBN: 978-1-138-91045-4 (pbk)
ISBN: 978-1-315-69342-2 (ebk)

Typeset in Bembo
by Florence Production Ltd, Stoodleigh, Devon, UK

MIX
Paper from
responsible sources
FSC® C013056

Printed and bound in Great Britain by
TJ International Ltd, Padstow, Cornwall

We, the editors, dedicate this book to Senior Constable Jennifer Barker (NSW Police Force, Australia); Di Macleod, Director of Gold Coast Center Against Sexual Violence (Australia); and Shannon Lambert-Cooper, President of Pandora's Aquarium (USA) for their immeasurable aid to survivors of IPSV. It is dedicated also to the excellent men in our lives: Ken Plummer, Charles Peck, and Simon Easteal.

# Contents

# Contributors

**David Adams, EdD,** is co-founder as well as Co-Director of Emerge, the first counseling program in the US for men who abuse women, established in 1977. Dr. Adams has led groups for men who batter, and conducted outreach to victims of abuse, for 36 years. He has led parenting education classes for fathers for 12 years. As one of the nation's leading experts on men who batter, he has conducted training of social service and criminal justice professionals in 45 states and 16 nations. He has published numerous articles and book chapters, and writes a featured blog on *The Huffington Post*. Dr. Adams is a Commissioner on the Massachusetts Governor's Council on Sexual and Domestic Violence and Director of the National Domestic Violence Risk Assessment and Management Training Project. His book, *Why do they kill? Men who murder their intimate partners,* was published by Vanderbilt University Press in 2007.

**Thomas P. Alongi, JD,** graduated from the University of Kansas School of Law in 1989, and has practiced family, juvenile, criminal, and civil asset forfeiture law at various times over the past 27 years. He served as an assistant Geary County Attorney in Junction City, Kansas (1990–2000), an assistant U.S. Attorney in Tucson (2000–2001), an assistant Tucson City Prosecutor (2002–2004), and an associate attorney in private practice with Davis Miles, PLLC (2004–2007), handling both criminal defense and family law. Between January 2007 and June 2014, Tom worked as a senior staff attorney at Community Legal Services in downtown Phoenix, focusing his represen-tation on survivors of intimate partner violence in family court. He is now a partner and owner at Alongi & Donovan Law in Tempe, Arizona. In addition to his law practice, Tom has regularly appeared as a facilitator on family law topics for the Arizona Foundation for Legal Services & Education in a variety of settings. Tom and his wife, Betsy, live in Phoenix. In his spare time, he plays horn with the Salt River Brass, La Forza Chamber Orchestra, and East Valley Millennial Choirs & Orchestras. He also plays baseball and ice hockey.

**Lundy Bancroft** has 25 years of experience specializing in interventions for abusive men and their families. He has authored four books in the field, including the United States' best-selling book on domestic violence, *Why Does He Do That?* and the national prize-winner, *The Batterer as Parent.* Lundy is the former Training Director of Emerge, the nation's first counseling program for men who batter, and was involved in more than 2,000 cases as counselor and clinical supervisor. He has also served extensively as a custody evaluator, child abuse investigator, and expert witness. Lundy appears across the continent as a presenter for court personnel, child protective workers, mental health providers, law enforcement officials, and other audiences. He is currently writing a play with Patrice Lenowitz about battered women's experiences with the child custody system, called *Forbidden to protect.* His latest book, *Daily wisdom for "Why does he do that?": Encouragement for women involved with angry and controlling men,* was published in 2015.

**Joseph A. Camilleri, PhD,** is an Associate Professor of Psychology at Westfield State University. He studies the etiology of interpersonal conflict, particularly sexual conflict in committed relationships, and is interested in the application of scientific research toward program development and evaluation. Dr. Camilleri is also Director of the graduate program in Forensic Mental Health Counseling.

**Anna Carline, LLB (Hons), LLM, PhD,** is a senior lecturer in law at the University of Leicester in the UK. Her main areas of expertise are criminal law, in particular violence against women and sexual offenses, and feminist/gender theory. She has published extensively on the issues of rape and sexual assault, domestic homicide, prostitution, and trafficking. Anna's most recent work includes a British Academy-funded project concerned with evaluating rape law reform, and a book with Professor Patricia Easteal, *Shades of grey – Domestic and sexual violence against women: Law reform and society,* published by Routledge in 2014.

**Mike Davis** is a Police Sergeant for the Vancouver, Washington Police Department. He has been a police officer since 1991, serving as a police officer in Illinois prior to relocating to Vancouver. Sergeant Davis worked with community partnerships and department resources to help establish the City of Vancouver's first Domestic Violence Unit, which was named Community Partnership Team of the Year by the Washington State Department of Corrections in 2009, and served as the first Domestic Violence Sergeant. In 2004 he was named Outstanding Law Enforcement Officer by the Clark County Prosecuting Attorney's Office for service to the victims of domestic violence. From 2006 until 2012, he supervised detectives and probation officers while he coordinated the city's response to domestic violence crimes. Sergeant Davis serves on the Clark County Domestic Violence/Sexual Assault Task Force, participates in the STOP

Grant, and served on the Washington State Attorney General's Advisory Board on Domestic Violence. Sergeant Davis has presented for various national organizations and events. He is the author of two book chapters, one on investigating domestic violence cases and the other on law-enforcement response to intimate partner sexual violence.

**Walter S. DeKeseredy, PhD,** is Anna Deane Carlson Endowed Chair of Social Sciences, Director of the Research Center on Violence, and Professor of Sociology at West Virginia University. He has published 23 books and more than 170 scientific journal articles and book chapters on violence against women and other social problems. In 2008, the Institute on Violence, Abuse and Trauma gave him the Linda Saltzman Memorial Intimate Partner Violence Researcher Award. He also jointly received the 2004 Distinguished Scholar Award from the American Society of Criminology's (ASC) Division on Women and Crime and the 2007 inaugural UOIT Research Excellence Award. In 1995, he received the Critical Criminologist of the Year Award from the ASC's Division on Critical Criminology (DCC) and in 2008 the DCC gave him the Lifetime Achievement Award. In 2014, he received the Critical Criminal Justice Scholar Award from the Academy of Criminal Justice Sciences' Section on Critical Criminal Justice, and in 2015 he received the Career Achievement Award from the ASC's Division on Victimology.

**Patricia Easteal, AM, PhD,** is a Professor of Law at the University of Canberra who describes herself as an academic, author, advocate, and activist. In 2010 she was awarded an Australian honor "for service to the community, education and the law through promoting awareness and understanding of violence against women, discrimination and access to justice for minority groups." The same year she was named the ACT Australian of the Year. She was a finalist in Australian Human Rights awards in 2012. She also received an ALTC Excellence Award for Teaching in 2008. She has published 16 books and more than 160 academic publications primarily focusing on access to justice for women. Her most recent books include *Shades of grey – Domestic and sexual violence against women: Law reform and society* (co-authored with Anna Carline) (Routledge, 2014).

**"Eleanor," Diploma of Teaching, Bachelor of Education, Masters of Teaching (DipBM).** Eleanor is the pseudonym for an advocate for women who have escaped violence and then faced the challenges of navigating their way through family law and criminal law proceedings. Eleanor founded an online support group for women facing adversity. In her advocacy she has drawn from the victims' experiences and represented the women who are unable to tell their stories directly due to family law restrictions. Eleanor is an educator who has centered her work in developing civics and citizenship through community-based learning and assisting students to develop positive relationships with members of their local community.

**Kathryn Ford, LCSW.** As Children and Families Specialist at the Center for Court Innovation, Kathryn provides training and technical assistance to state and tribal justice systems through both the Tribal Justice Exchange and the Domestic Violence, Sexual Violence and Family Court Programs team. This includes assisting with community needs assessment, development and dissemination of best practices, authoring publications, and providing support around justice program development and management. Kathryn Ford has published articles in *Sexual Assault Report, Family & Intimate Partner Violence Quarterly*, and the National Coalition Against Domestic Violence's *The Voice*; has authored several Center publications; and has conducted training workshops for more than 4,000 participants from multiple disciplines. She also provides trauma-focused therapy and court support services to children, teens and their caregivers through the Center's Child and Adolescent Witness Support Program, which is located at the Bronx District Attorney's Office, and is the Director of Clinical Supervision for the Center. Prior to joining the Center, Kathryn was a social worker in Safe Horizon's Supervised Visitation Program at Bronx Family Court and an intern in the Kings County District Attorney's Office's Counseling Services Unit. She received a Bachelor's degree in Psychology and Sociology from Tufts University and a Master's degree in Social Work from Columbia University, and is certified in Rape Crisis Counseling.

**Marie M. Fortune, MDiv, DHLet, DDiv,** is a pastor, author, educator, and practicing ethicist and theologian. She grew up in North Carolina, where she received her undergraduate degree from Duke University. She received her seminary training at Yale Divinity School and was ordained a minister in the United Church of Christ in 1976. After serving in a local parish, in 1977 Rev. Fortune founded FaithTrust Institute (www.faithtrustinstitute.org), a national, multifaith, multicultural organization providing religious communities and advocates with training, consultation, and educational materials to address the faith aspects of abuse. She was Editor of *The Journal of Religion and Abuse* from 2000 to 2008 and served on the National Advisory Council on Violence Against Women for the U.S. Department of Justice (1995–2000) and the Defense Task Force on Domestic Violence for the U.S. Department of Defense (2000–2003). She is the author of numerous books including *Sexual violence: The sin revisited* (1983, 2005) and *Keeping the faith: Guidance for Christian women facing abuse* (1987).

**Rus Ervin Funk, MSW,** is a community organizer and therapist who has been working to end gender-based violence since 1983, and to engage and organize men since 1987. He is the co-founder of DC Men Against Rape (now Men Can Stop Rape, Inc.), and numerous other organizations, including the Baltimore Alliance Against Child Sexual Abuse; Men for Gender Justice; Mobilizing to End violeNce (M.E.N.); MENSWORK: eliminating violence against women, inc.; the Ohio Men's Action Network; and the North American MenEngage Network (NAMEN). He is currently the Coordinator of Male Engagement for the Center for Women and Families, and facilitates the Own It Initiative (www.rusfunk.me). Rus serves on the Steering Committee of NAMEN and on the board of directors of the National Resource Center on Sexual and Domestic Violence. He also consults regularly throughout the U.S. and is recognized by the U.S. State Department to work with host countries to mobilize men in support of women's human rights. Rus has written numerous articles and chapters on issues related to engaging men, working with men, and preventing gender-based violence. Rus's first book, *Stopping rape: A challenge for men*, (1993) was the first book written by a man, for men, about stopping rape. His latest book, *Reaching men: Strategies for preventing sexist attitudes, behaviors and violence* (2004) is widely regarded as a critical resource for engaging men and boys. Rus lives in Louisville, KY, with his partner, their six-year-old child, and a cat who belongs to himself. He loves to cook, write, read, garden, photograph, and bike-ride.

**Liz Kelly, PhD (Sociology), BA (First Class, Sociology and Politics),** is Professor of Sexualised Violence at London Metropolitan University, where she is also director of the Child and Woman Abuse Studies Unit (CWASU). She has been active in the field of violence against women and children for almost 30 years. She is the author of *Surviving sexual violence* (1988), which established the concept of a "continuum of violence," and more than 70 book chapters and journal articles. Liz has completed a project looking at the trafficking of persons for both labor and sexual exploitation in Central Asia. In 2000 she was awarded a CBE in the New Year's Honours List for "services combating violence against women and children," and in January 2005 she was appointed to the Board of Commissioners of the Women's National Commission.

**Jennifer Y. Levy-Peck, PhD,** is a licensed psychologist and directs her own human services firm, Levy-Peck Consulting, LLC. She provides training and technical writing related to victim advocacy and related topics, and serves as the Accreditor for Washington State sexual assault programs. She is also a Training and Development Specialist for End Violence Against Women International. She formerly worked as Program Management Specialist for the Washington Coalition of Sexual Assault Programs. Dr. Levy-Peck has worked with trauma survivors and in program development for more than 30 years. She has written a book for parents of children who have been sexually abused, and has been a presenter at national, regional, and local conferences. She is co-editor (and has written several chapters) of *Intimate partner sexual violence: A multidisciplinary guide to improving services and support for survivors of rape and abuse*. She and her husband live among the evergreens in Washington State.

**Weiwei Liu, PhD,** is a criminologist at NORC at the University of Chicago. Dr. Liu's research covers the developmental etiology of risky and criminal behavior and evaluating intervention trials that target these behaviors. More specifically, Liu's research focuses on understanding the developmental risk factors of problem behavior and health consequences particularly in vulnerable populations, evaluating preventive intervention trials targeting youth violence, and evaluating interventions targeting substance use and mental health problems in high risk populations.

**Janet Loughman** is the Principal Solicitor at Women's Legal Service NSW where she has been for the past 10 years. She has worked as a solicitor initially in private practice and then in the community sector for over 25 years. Janet was awarded the NSW Justice Medal in 2005 for access to justice services to disadvantaged communities. In 2015 she appeared before the Royal Commission into Institutional Responses to Child Sexual Abuse in the Bethcar Case Study giving evidence about WLS's case for 13 Aboriginal women who took a breach of duty of care case against the state for its failure to protect them from abuse in care.

**Angela Lynch** is the community education and law reform lawyer at Women's Legal Service in Brisbane, and is currently the Queensland representative on the Women's Legal Services Australia coordinating committee. She has previously been the national law reform coordinator of Women's Legal Services Australia. Angela takes a lead role in the development of Women's Legal Service policy on legal reform issues at a state and national level, and she has successfully managed a number of key community education projects for the Service. Along with Associate Professor Rachael Field, she was one of the principal authors of the Coordinated Family Dispute Resolution (FDR) model, which was a specialized model of FDR developed for the Attorney-General's Department in 2011 for families who had experienced family violence.

**Louise McOrmond–Plummer, Assoc. Dip. Welfare,** is an Australian feminist who survived domestic violence which included repeated rape by a man who attempted to kill her. After gaining her freedom, she graduated from La Trobe University (Victoria) and has devoted more than 20 years to the study of intimate partner sexual violence (IPSV). Louise's specialization in this topic is internationally respected through her writing, interviews and presentations. Louise co-facilitates training workshops for professionals about appropriately responding to IPSV. She is sitemistress of Aphrodite Wounded (www.aphroditewounded.org), the first comprehensive online IPSV resource for survivors and professionals. Louise has co-authored/coedited two previous books on IPSV with Professor Patricia Easteal, AM, *Real rape, real pain: Help for women sexually assaulted by male partners* (2006) and second, with Professor Easteal and Dr. Jennifer Y. Levy Peck, *Intimate* *partner sexual violence: A multidisciplinary guide to improving services and support for survivors of rape and abuse* (2014). Louise has supported women who have experienced violence in various ways, including court support, counseling survivors of sexual and domestic violence in a community mental health setting which lead her supervisor to call her "gifted" in this area, and ten years as a moderator of Pandora's Aquarium, a celebrated online resource for survivors of rape and sexual assault. Louise is a research associate with West Virginia University Research Center on Violence, and is on the management committee of the Gold Coast Centre Against Sexual Violence. She has five children and a beloved husband currently recovering from cancer.

**Lindsey Mason** is the single mother of four children and also the lucky grandmother of a little girl and little boy. She currently lives in Luxembourg and works full-time, maintaining the online domestic violence survivor resource *Hidden hurt* (www.hiddenhurt.co.uk) since 2001. Apart from her personal experiences and years of listening to other survivors of domestic abuse, Lindsey has completed several abuse-related courses, holds counseling qualifications, and is a qualified Freedom Programme Facilitator. Lindsey has also contributed to the book by Patricia Easteal and Louise McOrmond-Plummer, *Real rape, real pain: Help for women sexually assaulted by male partners*.

**Melissa M. Miele, MA,** completed her degree in Forensic Mental Health Counseling at John Jay College of Criminal Justice in New York. She is currently working as a Correctional Counselor in a women's correctional center in Massachusetts, providing counseling services to inmates struggling with addiction and mental illness, specifically symptomology related to trauma such as sexual victimization between intimate partners. Melissa Miele has also worked as a therapist in a domestic violence clinic in New York City, providing treatment to court-ordered male domestic violence and stalking offenders. Her research has primarily focused on the evolutionary perspective of intimate partner violence, more specifically the relationship between physical and sexual violence, sexual jealousy, and characteristics of psychopathy.

**Kat Monusky, MS,** is the Prevention Program Coordinator with the Washington Coalition of Sexual Assault Programs. In this role she provides primary prevention training, technical assistance, and resource development to support the work of sexual assault programs across the state. Previously she worked as an advocate for victims of sexual and intimate partner violence in community and campus settings. She received her Master's degree in Sociology, as well as a certificate in Gender Violence Intervention, from Virginia Commonwealth University.

**Elizabeth A. Mumford, PhD, MHS,** is a social epidemiologist at NORC at the University of Chicago, a social science research organization that collects and analyzes data on key social issues. She received her doctorate in population dynamics from the Johns Hopkins University School of

Public Health. Dr. Mumford's research includes studies of the epidemiology and prevention of interpersonal and intimate aggressive behavior. Dr. Mumford also maintains an active research portfolio in tobacco epidemiology, tobacco control policies, and the relevant social ecology.

**Debra Parkinson, PhD,** is a social researcher, focusing on gender issues. Over the past two decades, she has researched intimate partner violence and rape, women's unequal access to the legal system, and gendered discrimination through the superannuation system. Since 2009, her research has focused on environmental justice, and gender and disaster. In 2015, Debra was awarded the Social and Political Sciences Graduate Research Thesis Award from Monash University for her doctoral work on increased domestic violence after the Victorian "Black Saturday" bushfires. She is currently an Adjunct Research Fellow with Monash University Disaster Resilience Initiative, and long-time researcher for both Women's Health in the North and Women's Health Goulburn North East.

**Evan Stark.** A founder of one of the first shelters for abused women in the U.S., Evan Stark is a sociologist and a forensic social worker as well as a widely published author and award-winning researcher with an international reputation for his innovative work on the legal, policy, and health dimensions of interpersonal violence. Professor Stark's award-winning book on *Coercive control* helped change the understanding and response to partner abuse in the US and the UK, and was an important basis for the new offense of "domestic violence and coercive control" in England and Wales. He is Emeritus Professor at Rutgers University in New Jersey and has also held appointments at Yale University, the University of Essex, Bristol University, and most recently was the Leverhulme Visiting Professor at the University of Edinburgh.

**Nan Stein, EdD,** is a senior research scientist at the Wellesley Centers for Women, where she directs several national research projects. For over 30 years, her research has focused on sexual harassment and teen dating violence in K-12 Schools, and she is the author of numerous book chapters and articles published in law review journals and scholarly journals, as well as op-ed pieces in the mainstream press and curriculum materials for schools. She frequently gives lectures, keynote addresses, and training to school personnel, and serves as an expert witness in lawsuits on sexual harassment and child sexual abuse in K-12 schools. Dr. Stein was Co-PI for the Shifting Boundaries experiments.

**Bruce G. Taylor, PhD, Senior Fellow, NORC,** at the University of Chicago, has more than 20 years of experience in applied research and evaluation, with specific expertise in research design, measurement, survey design, and analysis. Dr. Taylor's research covers the areas of victimization and the broader field of conducting violence prevention research, youth violence, teen dating violence, victim services, and policing research. As a criminologist, he has focused on identifying demographic and contextual explanations for a variety of forms of violent behaviors and related risky behaviors. Dr. Taylor has led more than a dozen randomized experiments covering a variety of public safety/public health topics and has conducted longitudinal research regarding intimate partner violence (IPV) and other topical areas. His work in the area of victimization dates back to the 1990s, when he was researching the psychological recovery process of rape victims recruited from rape crisis centers and emergency rooms in New York City.

**Nicole Westmarland, PhD,** is Professor of Criminology at Durham University where she is Director of the Durham Centre for Research into Violence and Abuse (CRiVA). She was previously Chair of Rape Crisis (England and Wales) and continues to be a trustee of her local Rape Crisis Centre. Her most recent book is *Violence against women: Criminological perspectives on men's violences* (Routledge, 2015).

# Foreword

The subjects of this comprehensive, well-researched, and disturbing collection are the men who have sexually assaulted a partner (intimate partner sexual violence, or IPSV) and the effects on the women and children who are victimized by them. Internationally renowned authors joined by survivors present original research, practical experience, and first-person narratives to examine the prevalence, dynamics, consequences, societal significance, sources, and best ways to prevent IPSV. The book is long overdue, much needed, and path-breaking.

As I write, U.S. media are highlighting a petition signed by over one million people to recall a California judge because he sentenced a student to *only* six months for raping a woman in a drunken stupor. The perpetrator was also drunk, a star athlete, and testified that the victim seemed to be enjoying herself, though she didn't remember what happened and two witnesses testified she was unconscious. A decade ago, a case with these facts would not have been prosecuted, let alone resulted in conviction. Even today, there is almost no chance the case would have gone to trial had the victim and assailant been middle-age intimates instead of youthful strangers. I am writing this from Belfast, Northern Ireland, where the High Court just upheld only the country's third conviction for marital rape since 1990, when the behavior was made an offense.

Despite the fact that male partners comprise the largest class of rape offenders, including those reported to police, they remain largely invisible to the justice and legal systems as well as to researchers who specialize in rape. In the UK, partners are eight times more likely than strangers to be reported to police for rape (31% vs. 3.8%). Yet just slightly more than 3 in 100 of these reported offenders is convicted of a crime, usually a lesser offense (Hester & Westmarland, 2006). Unlike stranger rapes, where assailants are often hard to locate, intimate partners are readily accessible. Thus, if perpetrators of IPSV are invisible to the community at large, they are also in plain sight.

I became aware of the significance of IPSV in the early 1980s, a decade before marital rape became a crime in the U.S. and U.K. As part of the Yale Trauma Studies that Anne Flitcraft and I co-directed on how domestic violence affected women's health, Roper reviewed the medical records of the 174 rape victims who had used Yale–New Haven Hospital in the previous two years. The findings frame my appreciation of this collection.

Battered women comprised 18% of the patient population in our larger sample. However, they accounted for 50% of the rapes ever reported by women (Stark & Flitcraft, 1996). Among the subsample of rape victims, meanwhile, approximately one in three had a documented history of battering and 58% of the rape victims over 30 were battered women (Roper, Flitcraft, & Frazier, 1979). Moreover, during abusive histories that lasted 7.2 years on average, the battered rape victims had often reported multiple sexual assaults, anticipating the later finding that IPSV accounts for a far higher proportion of rapes than it does for rape victims. Much of the physical violence these women suffered was also sexual, with injuries clustering around their face, breasts, and abdomen.

These preliminary findings suggested two facts documented throughout this volume: that partners rather than strangers are the typical men who rape women and that woman battering is the typical context for IPSV. According to government statistics, partners and strangers respectively account for 56%, and 8% of reported rapes in Australia; 45.4% and 11% in the UK; and 51% and 13% in the U.S. Because IPSV is reported far less often than stranger rape, the actual ratios of partner/stranger rape are far higher. This fact also demystifies a claim often used to discredit IPSV victims, that most men who rape are "known" by their victims. Subsequent research has also confirmed the point emphasized by Davis (Chapter 19), that assessments of domestic violence must include IPSV. Some 40–60% of the battered women who seek outside assistance report they have been sexually assaulted; 27% report being "forced to have sex against their will" "often" or "all the time" and 24% report being forced to engage in anal sex at least once (Rees, Agnew-Davies, & Barkham, 2006).

To these conclusions, another must be added – that the type of battering most closely associated with IPSV is *coercive control*, a pattern of abuse in which the repeated physical and sexual violence is accompanied by some combination of threats, stalking, and other forms of *intimidation* and tactics designed to degrade, *isolate* and *control* partners by exploiting them as servants, depriving them of money and other vital resources, and regulating their everyday lives (Stark, 2007). According to a recent random population survey by the U.S. Centers for Disease Control and Prevention, for example, 85% of the women who reported a rape by a partner had also been physically assaulted and/or stalked (Black et al., 2011). "Louise," in Chapter 5, highlights how intimidation and control provided the context for IPSV in her life:

> In six years I wasn't allowed to have any money, I wasn't allowed to drive a car, everywhere I went he went with me and I wasn't allowed out of the house, and if I didn't answer the phone he would be on the doorstep within an hour saying "Where were you?" So there was huge control, huge control.

Importantly, 15% of partner rape victims report that IPSV was the only form of physical abuse they experienced, a finding illustrated by Lindsay Mason's testimony (Chapter 9).

Another relevant finding from the Yale research was a marked disconnect between the Rape Protocol followed by the hospital's Rape Crisis Intervention Team (RCIT) and victims' perception of their needs. The Protocol anticipated that women had experienced sexual assault as a trauma outside the realm of their normal experience; traced behaviors such as changing locks or fear of returning home or going outside to "rape trauma syndrome"; urged them to cooperate with prosecution; and attempted to "normalize" their experience by sharing it with significant others such as husbands or boyfriends. When victims of IPSV responded negatively to this protocol, they were given victim-blaming labels that suggested they were not "real" rape victims and so not entitled to full support. The RCIT attributed this "failure" to fit the conventional rape profile to the fact that IPSV victims often had histories of multiple victimizations and/or suffered from psychological and/or behavioral problems such as depression or substance abuse. In the eyes of the RCIT, these women were prone to victimization *because* of their problematic histories. Ironically, these same factors – failure to cooperate (by dropping charges, for example), repeat reports of rape and behavioral problems – underlie the decisions by police and prosecution not to charge IPSV offenders (Hester, 2006).

A number of chapters in this book trace the poor reception of perpetrators and victims of IPSV to the propensity to interpret their behavior/experience through the prism of myths of "real" (i.e. stranger) rape and make their "resistance" intelligible as a byproduct of their ongoing predicament. IPSV victims often drop charges because their assailants are still in the home or community; they experience sexual assault as part of the ongoing pattern of abuse noted by Adams (Chapter 1) rather than as an isolated trauma; and they abuse substances or become depressed in the process of coping with coercive control, an adaptive process I term "control in the context of no control." Far from being maladaptive, cautions such as changing locks or refusing to return home are rational steps to avoid ongoing abuse, even if they are not always effective. Reframing based on the specificity of IPSV could ensure a far better reception of victims.

Perpetrators of IPSV also "fail" tests set to identify typical rapists, though this benefits rather than hurts their prospects. The medico–legal narrative portrays rapists as disadvantaged violence-prone men who are isolated from peers; unable to form stable or long-term relationships; suffer a variant of sociopathy, psychopathy or a related personality disorder; and are driven to sexual assault by some combination of childhood trauma, wounded masculinity, and/or misogyny. Several chapters in this volume identify commonalities among all men who rape, such as a propensity for pornography. Nonetheless, without the training outlined by Westmarland and Kelly (Chapter 18) and Davis (Chapter 19) that challenges rape myths and links the vulnerability to IPSV of women like Louise to the fact that they are being threatened, degraded, isolated and controlled, all involved weigh women's allegations as wanting compared to the Mr. Normal Nice Guy described by his family, co-workers, pals, and court evaluators.

The myth that "real" rape is a choice rooted in psychopathology can lead Family Courts to excuse a certain amount of physical/sexual abuse as "situational," e.g. as provoked by jealousy or the threat of separation, and to side with a perpetrator in a custody dispute, particularly after their cross-examination of a frightened partner shows her to be confused, friendless, uncooperative, and obsessed with accusations for which there is often no corroboration.

As any important scholarly collection should do, this volume challenges conventional thinking in the field without honing to a single "best" approach. One challenge involves where to situate IPSV heuristically so as to mount the most effective strategies for intervention and prevention. Should we continue to view IPSV as one among several types of rape, place it on the spectrum of sexual coercion identified with coercive control, or view it through the lens of a culture of masculinity and hetero-normativity into which most men are socialized? Advocates of the "rape is rape" approach want an identical justice response regardless of the context of sexual assault (Raphael, 2013) while emphasizing normative masculinity suggests a combination of preventative gender re-education and innovative counseling initiatives (Chapters 17, 18, and 21).

Setting IPSV in the context of coercive control means pursuing partner rapes as part of a criminal pattern as Britain has done by creating a new offense of "domestic violence and coercive control." These approaches suggest very different ways to invest scarce resources.

Defining marital rape as a crime was a major step in women's self-governance, challenged the common law understanding of rape as a violation of patriarchal property rights to women's bodies, and lifted the veil that had insulated "private" offenses against women from public law. However, apart from their proximate physical similarities, the gender identity of typical perpetrators/victims and the importance of inequality-based patriarchal privilege in all violence against women (VAW), stranger rape and IPSV have little in common. The perpetrators and victims have different psychological and behavioral profiles and demographic characteristics. Stranger rape and IPSV occur in different settings; derive from different motives; incur different experiences of violation; and involve different risks of repeat, injurious, and/or fatal physical/sexual assault, stalking or other crimes. Research in this volume shows that some of these differences are better established than others. Even so, their phenomenological differences mean that framing IPSV as "rape" is a strategic choice. I worry that the singular advantage of demanding serious sanctions for intimate partners can be outweighed by the extent to which the "rape is rape" approach throws the normative nature of IPSV and its typical context into the shadows.

The victim voices heard throughout this book suggest that IPSV is "lived" as a dimension of sexual coercion and coercive control. Forced pregnancies and abortions, sabotage of birth control and the other forms of "reproductive coercion" by which IPSV perpetrators maintain power and control over reproductive health are brilliantly elucidated in Chapter 11. These insults occur on a continuum of sexual coercion that extends to sexual inspections, sex trafficking, exposure to pornography and "rape as routine," perhaps the most common form of sexual exploitation, where women comply with their partner's sexual demands because of the "or else" proviso. As one woman reported to Easteal and McOrmond-Plummer:

> The best way I can describe it is that there was an unspoken threat that if I didn't have sex with him he would emotionally abuse me. He would throw a tantrum if I said no, guilt trip me. Ignore me, reject me, and because he had convinced me that I was in love with him and couldn't live without him these things hurt me a lot so in a way, I submitted to sex because it was the only way to avoid emotional/mental pain.
>
> (cited in Chapter 4)

This woman's vulnerability to sexual exploitation is a function of a pattern of intimidation and psychological abuse that is only distally linked to the rape chronology, making it hard to prove the elements of "rape." But the absence of force does not diminish the loss of dignity and autonomy replicated by the sex act, making a mockery of legal approaches that equate compliance or lack of resistance with consent. If setting IPSV in the context of coercive control diminishes some of the stigma attached to rapists, it reframes compliance, repeat or withdrawn complaints, secondary problems and other facets of IPSV used to discredit women's allegations of rape as evidence that sexual coercion occurred, greatly facilitating prosecution and convictions whether the rape(s) is charged in addition to or as part of coercive control. Viewing IPSV through the prism of coercive control also highlights its political dimension as a violation of women's civil and human rights and the importance for prevention of embracing the equality agenda alongside a more robust justice response.

The sheer prevalence of IPSV highlights the greatest challenge posed by designing a response to IPSV: how to reconcile individually based interventions for behaviors enacted by tens of millions of men. Great care must be taken not to adapt the perspective of the male perpetrators Adams interviewed (Chapter 1) who "normalized" their violence. And yet, there is no way to avoid the conclusion that IPSV is a social fact rooted in normative structures that misallocate rights, privileges, and resources according to sexual identity, and which helps sustain heteronormativity as a socioeconomic and cultural system of male entitlement. In this volume, Parkinson, DeKeseredy, Bancroft, McOrmond-Plummer and others dissect the "normative masculinity" expressed through IPSV, echoing Connell's (2005) insistence that any challenge to "hegemonic" masculinity must include support for alternative and nonhegemonic masculinities which draw power from respect and equality with other men and women.

Whether or not we regard "patriarchy" as a useful concept, the persistent treatment of women's bodies as male property must be addressed in its social context, not merely as a set of attitudes or beliefs, including the class and race-based networks and hierarchies men establish among themselves and through which they control other men as well as women and children. These include the "hyper-erotic" networks DeKeseredy examines that men establish in cyberspace and which fuel men's anger by creating expectations about sex that cannot be met. The importance of social context is illustrated by the requirement by Men Stopping Violence in Atlanta, Georgia (described in Chapter 17) that a perpetrator's peers be included in counseling. Several stories in the book also illustrate how women can also be entrapped by male gender ideology, as when they submit to IPSV as part of their marital "obligation" or feel religion requires them to marry men who raped them, a dilemma Fortune addresses (Chapter 16).

I am convinced by this volume that our responses to VAW would be greatly enhanced by a reconceptualization of rape centered on IPSV. At a minimum, such a reconceptualization would highlight the prevalence and distinctiveness of IPSV; the inextricable relationship to other forms of coercion and control; its roots in normative/hegemonic masculinity; and the extent to which the justice and legal systems would be improved by substituting an evidence-based understanding of IPSV for medico-legal images of "real" rape and rapists. Conversely, based on data from *Project Mirabel*, Westmarland and Kelly (Chapter 18) observe that programs designed for sexual predators/rapists are not appropriate for men who commit sexual assault in the context of coercive control. A concurrent reassessment is needed to highlight the importance of IPSV in domestic violence and coercive control.

Carline and Easteal (Chapter 15) argue persuasively that courts should broaden their criteria for vitiating consent requirements in IPSV cases to include the forms of intimidation that occur in intimate relationships. If dictums such as "affirmative consent" already give more weight to the alleged rapist's opinion of whether consent was given than is merited by women's right to control their bodies, the case examples in this volume illustrate that compliance is never voluntary in the context of coercive control.

In the common law understanding of rape as violating the property rights of fathers and husbands, IPSV was a contradiction in terms. Exposing IPSV to public scrutiny is a major step toward reclaiming for women what is rightfully theirs. But the "personal is political," as the old feminist adage has it. The suffering of IPSV victims can only be ended when steps to hold perpetrators fully to account are coupled with a human rights agenda of equality, dignity, and liberty for all, men as well as women and children.

*Evan Stark*

# References

Black, M.C., Basile, K.C., Breiding, M.J., Smith, S.G., Walters, M.L., Merrick, M.T., Chen, J., & Stevens, M.R. (2011). *The National Intimate Partner and Sexual Violence Survey (NISVS): 2010 Summary Report.* Atlanta, GA: National Center for Injury Prevention and Control, Centers for Disease Control.

Connell, R.W. (2005). *Masculinities* (2nd ed.). Berkeley, CA: University of California Press.

Hester, M. (2006). Making it through the criminal justice system: Attrition and domestic violence. *Social Policy and Society, 5*(1), 1–12.

Hester, M. & Westmarland, N. (2006). Domestic violence perpetrators. *Criminal Justice Matters, 66*(1), 34–35.

Raphael, J. (2013). *Rape is rape: How denial, distortion and victim blaming are fueling a hidden acquaintance rape crisis.* Chicago, IL: Lawrence Hill Books.

Rees, A., Agnew-Davies, R., & Barkham, M. (2006, June). Outcomes for women escaping domestic violence at refuge. Paper presented at the Society for Psychotherapy Research Annual Conference, Edinburgh, UK.

Roper, M., Flitcraft, A., & Frazier, W. (1979). *Rape and battering.* Unpublished paper. Department of Surgery. Yale Medical School.

Stark, E. (2007). *Coercive control: How men entrap women in personal life.* New York, NY: Oxford University Press.

Stark, E., & Flitcraft, A. (1996). *Women at risk: Domestic violence and women's health.* Thousand Oaks, CA: Sage.

# Acknowledgments

We are grateful to all of the chapter authors for their contributions. They were chosen for their varied fields of expertise and experience, and their common passion for justice. In addition, we thank Louisa Vahtrick and Shannon Kneis for their guidance throughout the publication process. Special thanks go to the survivors of intimate partner sexual violence who have courageously shared their thoughts and experiences throughout this book, and to professionals who are working to change the way that communities and nations address sexual violence. Lastly, what might appear obvious – our gratitude to each other. We have each had particularly challenging experiences during the gestational period of this book. However, through sheer determination and our ties as "sisters," we have taken turns at ensuring the completion of this important book to help those working with IPSV to better understand perpetrators. Information is power and the fertile ground for change.

# Part 1

# Moving the focus to perpetrators and their impact

# Chapter 1

# Introduction

## Why a focus on perpetrators of intimate partner sexual violence is essential

*Louise McOrmond-Plummer, Patricia Easteal, and Jennifer Y. Levy-Peck*

The burgeoning literature of the past several decades about perpetrators of rape and sexual assault has focused mostly on convicted stranger rapists and those who sexually abuse children (Greathouse, Saunders, Matthews, Keller, & Miller, 2015). Most discourse on perpetrators of sexual assault excludes men who rape and sexually assault their intimate partners. This contributes to widely held beliefs that only stranger rapists are *real* rapists, while at the same time those beliefs shape research topics. Social awareness campaigns instruct girls and women to beware the stranger, and how to avoid sexual assault by watching how much or with whom they drink (see, for example, Baty, 2014). The reality, however, is that intimate partner sexual assault (IPSV) has been established as a prevalent crime since the 1980s. Intimate relationships in fact comprise a far greater danger of sexual assault to women (Black et al., 2011; Finkelhor & Yllo, 1990; Myhill & Allen, 2002; Price, 2013; Russell, 1985). Limited focus on these perpetrators ensures a persistent avoidance of detection and accountability, and ongoing danger to women.

Therefore, the partner rapist is seldom recognized as a rapist or sexual offender in the same sense as a stranger rapist or pedophile, even though the rape of a spouse has been a criminal act in the Western world for a number of decades. Further, the majority of partner rapists do not see their behavior as criminal (Parkinson & Cowan, 2008). The same view is upheld by many in the criminal justice system, with particularly low levels of prosecution and conviction (see Chapter 14).

Yet IPSV may result in longer term effects than stranger rape (Finkelhor & Yllo, 1985; Russell, 1990). IPSV perpetrators frequently inflict higher levels of physical violence than perpetrators of rape in other contexts (Myhill & Allen, 2002). Further, it is vital to learn more about perpetrators of IPSV because batterers who also rape are more likely to kill, as discussed in the following chapter. While IPSV is a common behavior of perpetrators of physical violence (Black et al., 2011), it is also committed by men who do not necessarily batter their partners. They may not even use physical force to negate consent, instead using a range of coercive tactics such as withdrawing affection or withholding housekeeping money, not allowing their partner to sleep, or repeatedly badgering her to engage in acts she has stated she does not like (Easteal & McOrmond-Plummer, 2006). Sexual activity enacted with this sort of duress is rape/sexual assault.

It is important that people who work in relevant occupations learn more about these types of IPSV perpetrators. This includes but is not limited to counselors, police, batterer group facilitators, and youth workers. People in the community, including students (both undergraduate and graduate), survivors, and others could benefit from learning more about these hidden offenders. However, this book is not enough. More research is needed on IPSV.

We hope that the current work provides direction for further investigation and intervention. For instance, the focus of this volume is male-on-female perpetration of IPSV. Our language will reflect this, with female pronouns for victims, and male pronouns for perpetrators, although we recognize that victims and offenders may be of other genders. Readers should also be aware, though, that this form of victimization may occur in same-sex relationships (Ristock, 2014). Even less is known about this group of perpetrators, and we hope to see further research in this direction. Another group not included in this book but certainly deserving of inquiry are older perpetrators of IPSV. Their victims may be especially vulnerable if the perpetrator is their caregiver, or because of cognitive impairments that impact on the perception of their credibility (Ramsey-Klawsnik & Brandl, 2009).

## What this book contains

### Part 1: Moving the focus to perpetrators and their impact

Much of the literature on gender-based violence focuses on survivors, because they are more likely than perpetrators to be cooperative research subjects. In Part 1, we shift the focus to perpetrators and, beginning with the current chapter, explain why it is so important to understand who they are and what they do. David Adams is an expert who has interviewed men who murdered their partners. He gives valuable insight into why batterers who rape, kill their partners more frequently than batterers who do not rape, and why it is important to identify IPSV in danger assessments in order to keep women safe. In examining what perpetrators do to those closest to them, we wanted to ensure that the impact of IPSV on children was clearly highlighted. Kathryn Ford discusses the effect of children's exposure to IPSV and their increased risk of direct sexual assault by these offenders.

### Part 2: Who are the perpetrators of intimate partner sexual violence?

Many people still confuse IPSV with sex, rather than the act of violence or control that it is. Patricia Easteal and Louise McOrmond-Plummer provide a look into the mindset of IPSV perpetrators, discussing their motivations, the myths that they may subscribe to in order to justify sexual violence, and the ways that they may avoid taking responsibility.

When men go through batterer treatment, discussing sexual violence could be a key trigger point for them to understand their behaviors as violent and abusive. Nicole Westmarland and Liz Kelly draw on interviews with men who have attended domestic violence perpetrator programs and look at the ways in which they talk about their use of sexual violence. Deb Parkinson also seeks to identify perpetrators' perceptions. In her 2008 study of IPSV, none of the perpetrators viewed acts of sexual assault as criminal – or indeed as rape. In her chapter, she looks at the deeply entrenched sense of entitlement that underpins perpetrators' lack of recognition, and how it may be challenged.

Joseph Camilleri and Melissa Miele explain that understanding the characteristics, conditions, typology, and motivations of IPSV perpetrators can guide those who are designing intervention programs. They believe in the value of accurate categorization and exploration of individual differences in psychological profiles. They argue that IPSV perpetrators constitute a diverse group whose treatment needs are distinct from those of other domestic abusers or sexual offenders.

Louise McOrmond-Plummer explores and challenges stereotypes of men who rape and the women who are raped, and how these preconceived notions can create barriers when working with perpetrators or their victims. Because IPSV takes place within a relationship, understanding relationship dynamics may be quite useful. This chapter explores additional factors that may bind women to perpetrators (Holmes & Holmes, 2009), without detracting from the seriousness of the crime.

### Part 3: Perpetrators' strategies for control

We believe it is important to look at IPSV, like other forms of partner violence, as a mechanism for coercive control (Stark, 2007). In Part 3, we describe the specific means that IPSV perpetrators use to maintain that control. Louise McOrmond-Plummer explores the various strategies that perpetrators of IPSV may use to force or coerce their partners into sexual activity. This chapter will aid practitioners in understanding both the physically violent and nonviolent forms of IPSV, and sets the stage for the next two chapters, which look more in depth at these different types of IPSV perpetrating.

Indeed, although IPSV is committed most often by perpetrators who also use physical violence, there are partner rapists who do not batter. This is important for professionals to know about; many continue to see rape as necessarily involving additional physical violence. Survivor and domestic violence activist Lindsey Mason draws a picture of her victimization by a perpetrator who, though he did not beat her, raped her so frequently that she experienced medical problems as a result. Then Louise McOrmond-Plummer discusses her experience of a battering partner rapist: the characteristics, potential lethality, and the situations that tended to fuel sexually violent behavior.

Perpetrators may further exert control by limiting their partners' reproductive choices or interfering with their reproductive health. Jennifer Y. Levy-Peck describes how various forms of reproductive coercion fit into the spectrum of abusive behaviors, including interference with birth control and other childbearing decisions.

### Part 4: How perpetrators are condoned: the social context of intimate partner sexual violence

The harms of IPSV and the criminality of its perpetrators are so often minimized. This does not take place in a vacuum. Part 4 looks at the contributory role of cultural factors and attitudes which make the degradation of women acceptable. And, holistically, social institutions such as the law and religion may support the perpetrator of IPSV.

Walter S. DeKeseredy has studied the phenomenon of male support of perpetrators as an important factor in IPSV. He explores themes such as what peer compliance looks like, and how it can be challenged socially and professionally. Following that chapter, he and Rus Ervin Funk discuss the degradation of women via pornography and how this may translate into degradation of women in intimate relationships by male pornography consumers. They present data from interviews with IPSV survivors who have experienced that direct link to pornography.

The response of the criminal justice system is an important component in the social context of IPSV. Anna Carline and Patricia Easteal examine ways in which police, prosecutors, and the courts continue to fail to see IPSV as "real rape." They provide recommendations for how the criminal justice system can improve the response to IPSV perpetrators. While most IPSV cases are not prosecuted in criminal court (as indeed, very few sexual assaults make it through the court system), family courts are more likely to become involved. The chapter on family law, co-authored by two lawyers and a survivor, highlights how family courts are not designed to ensure the safety of victims. Indeed, other research has found that judges often see sexual assault as immaterial when granting visitation or custody to abusers (Schafran, 2014). Angela Lynch, Janet Loughman, and survivor "Eleanor" show how IPSV perpetrators are able to manipulate the family court system and be supported by that system. Tom Alongi's commentary within this chapter expands the scope to family law in the U.S., and the chapter contains recommendations for change.

Religious communities provide another type of institutional response to IPSV. Marie Fortune discusses IPSV perpetrators in communities of faith, and ways of ensuring that faith communities hold perpetrators responsible. This chapter also describes how the three major faith traditions – Islam, Judaism, and Christianity – expressly forbid sexual abuse of partners.

## Part 5: Community prevention and intervention with perpetrators

This section of the book focuses on remedies. These chapters provide ways for social institutions and individuals to intervene with and work more effectively with perpetrators, and also to help decrease IPSV. Rus Ervin Funk and Lundy Bancroft, who work with violent men, give strategies for addressing IPSV as part of the treatment of batterers. They describe methods for breaking down abuser denial and fostering a sense of responsibility.

As noted above, very few IPSV perpetrators face the criminal justice system. In the next chapter, police sergeant Mike Davis offers practical guidance for better identification of sexual crimes in domestic violence scenarios, dealing with IPSV suspects during the investigation and arrest process, and improving outcomes with respect to the victims.

Different paths to prevention are examined in the next chapters. For instance, can prevention be facilitated through education or awareness campaigns? Traditional sexual assault prevention has focused on teaching girls and women to keep themselves safe, yet effective prevention must begin with fundamental changes in community and societal attitudes, clear education about the nature of consent, and strategies for bystander involvement. Kat Monusky and Jennifer Y. Levy-Peck focus on true primary prevention of IPSV with young people, discussing effective ways of conceptualizing and addressing the roots of IPSV, and offering suggested best practices for prevention.

Turning to the classroom, Bruce Taylor, Elizabeth Mumford, Weiwei Lu, and Nan Stein share the results of a follow-up study on *Shifting Boundaries,* the evidence-based primary prevention program for middle-school students on sexual harassment and precursors to teen dating violence. This program has been recognized by the White House and the U.S. Centers for Disease Control and Prevention.

In the Conclusion, the editors extract and distill recommendations from the multidisciplinary, international experts who have contributed to this volume. The authors are a diverse group. Each has distinct viewpoints, which are not necessarily shared by other contributors or the editors. We do hope that the issues they raise will engender vital conversations among our readers. This book – a compilation of the scholarly and the experiential with a broader focus on violence against women juxtaposed with more narrow focus on IPSV – advances our knowledge of IPSV perpetration and how we, as professionals and members of our communities, can work to end this form of sexual violence.

## References

Baty, K. (2014, July 28). College freshman "must have" safety tips: It's ALL about the game plan [web log]. Retrieved from: http://safetychick.com/college-freshman-must-have-safety-tips-its-all-about-the-game-plan/.

Black, M.C., Basile, K.C., Breiding, M.J., Smith, S.G., Walters, M.L., Merrick, M.T., Chen, J., & Stevens, M.R. (2011). *The National Intimate Partner and Sexual Violence Survey (NISVS): 2010 Summary Report*. Atlanta, GA: National Center for Injury Prevention and Control, Centers for Disease Control and Prevention.

Easteal, P., & McOrmond-Plummer, L. (2006). *Real rape, real pain: Help for women sexually assaulted by male partners*. Melbourne, Australia: Hybrid Publishers.

Finklehor, D., & Yllo, K. (1985). *License to rape: Sexual abuse of wives*. New York, NY: The Free Press.

Greathouse, S.M., Saunders, J., Matthews, M., Keller, K.M., & Miller, L.L. (2015). A review of the literature on sexual assault perpetrator characteristics and behaviors. RAND Research Report. Retrieved from: www.rand.org/pubs/research_reports/RR1082.html.

Holmes, R.M., & Holmes, S.T. (2002). Psychological profiling and rape. In R.M. Holmes & S.T. Holmes (Eds.), *Profiling violent crimes: An investigative tool* (3rd ed.) (pp. 139–157). Thousand Oaks, CA: Sage.

Myhill, A., & Allen, J. (2002). Rape and sexual assault of women: Findings from the British Crime Survey. Retrieved from: www.aphroditewounded.org/Myhill%20and%20Allen.pdf.

Parkinson, D., & Cowan, S. (2008). *Raped by a partner: Nowhere to go, no-one to tell*. Victoria, Australia: Women's Goulburn North East.

Price, J. (2013, October 29). Sexual assault, too often, begins in the home. *The Canberra Times*. Retrieved from: www.canberratimes.com.au/comment/sexual-assault-too-often-begins-in-the-home-20131028–2wc1v.html.

Ramsey-Klawsnik, H., & Brandl, B. (2009, July/August). Sexual abuse in later life. *Sexual Assault Report*. Retrieved from: www.ncall.us/sites/ncall.us/files/resources/SAR1206-SA2-SexualAbuseLaterinLife.pdf.

Ristock, J. (2014). Sexual assault in intimate same-sex relationships. In L. McOrmond-Plummer, P. Easteal, & J. Levy-Peck (Eds.), *Intimate partner sexual violence: A multidisciplinary guide to improving services and support for survivors of rape and abuse* (pp. 259–269). London, UK: Jessica Kingsley Publishers.

Russell, D. (1990). *Rape in marriage*. Bloomington, IN: Indiana University Press.

Schafran, L.H. (2014). Intimate partner sexual violence and the courts. In L. McOrmond-Plummer, P. Easteal, & J. Levy-Peck (Eds.), *Intimate partner sexual violence: A multidisciplinary guide to improving services and support for survivors of rape and abuse* (pp. 221–233). London, UK: Jessica Kingsley Publishers.

Stark, E. (2007). *Coercive control: How men entrap women in personal life*. Oxford, UK: Oxford University Press.

# Chapter 2

# Talking to killers
## What can they tell us about sexual assault as a risk factor for homicide?

*David Adams*

## Sexual dynamics and lethality

Belying their minimizing and braggadocio, perpetrators of intimate partner homicides unwittingly provide useful information about the interconnections between sex and violence within the context of an abusive relationship. Their expectations about sex, and how they go about meeting these, provide retrospective insight into when and why sexual assaults unfold over time, and how they contribute to homicide. Sexual assault is a known risk factor for intimate partner homicide, but little is known about the specific ways that it intermeshes with other risk factors – such as threats to kill, estrangement, stalking, and extreme jealousy – that would appear to provide more straightforward pathways to murder (Campbell, Webster, Koziol-McLain, & McFarlane, 2003; Dobash & Dobash, 2015). Do sexual assaults provide a motive for killing? Or are they simply one additional element of the abuser's repertoire of abuse? Are sexual assaults more about sexual obsession or possession? What role do sexual assaults play in the abuser's attempts to control his partner? Moreover, *how specifically* do sexual assaults work as tactics of control? And are they effective?

To address these questions, I asked victims of attempted homicide and men who had killed their intimate partners to recount any instances of sexual assault that had occurred leading up to the killings and near-killings, and how these related to other events in the relationship. I was hoping that my questions about when and how sexual assaults occurred would help to clarify *why* they occurred. These questions were asked as part of a larger study about intimate partner homicides and attempted homicides that included in-depth interviews of 31 men who killed their partners as well as 20 women whose partners had tried to kill them (Adams, 2007).

Extensive semi-structured interviews of four to five hours' duration were conducted with the men who had killed. These interviews included taking a history of their relationship with the women they killed and also of their relationships with prior intimate partners. As part of this history, the men were asked to detail any abusive or controlling behavior they had committed, including what led up to it and its aftermath. Several measures were used to assess the frequency of abusive and controlling behaviors, including sexual violence and coercion. As additional sources of information about prior abusive behavior, I had access to the killers' criminal records, police reports, and, in some cases, trial transcripts and treatment records. Additional tools were used to assess the perpetrators' jealousy, perceived beliefs about women in general, and their attitudes toward their victims in particular.

Victims of attempted homicide were interviewed as "stand-ins" for murder victims who could not tell their own stories. It was important to include victims' perspectives as a counterpoint to the accounts of perpetrators, which have been found by various research studies to be self-serving and minimizing of their abusive behavior (Dobash & Dobash, 1979, Gondolf, 2002). My experience working with abusive men for more than 35 years, including outreach to their partners throughout the abuser's participation in treatment, has shown that there is almost always a substantial discrepancy between what the abuser reports and what the victim reports, with the latter reporting greater frequency and more severity in the violence. Over time with treatment, this discrepancy often lessens for many program participants as they begin to report more of their abusive behavior (Adams & Cayouette, 2002).

For the victims of attempted homicide, a semi-structured interview of four to six hours' duration was conducted. Each victim was asked to give a detailed chronology of her relationship with the offender, including how they met, what abusive and controlling behavior, if any, she had experienced, what seemed to trigger it, what her partner's most common grievances had been, and how her partner's behavior had changed over time. In addition to the interviews, victims were asked to complete several domestic violence assessment tools.

One of the major findings of the larger study, based on interviews with both victims and perpetrators, was that the triggers for the perpetrator's final assaults were not new motives but appeared to be a culmination of their longstanding grievances toward their partners, whether they were jealous accusations, complaints about money, or, in the case of those with alcohol problems, mundane grievances that arose on a daily basis (Adams, 2007).

## Chronologies of abuse

I asked each victim whether she had noticed any changes in her partner's abusive behavior during the course of their relationship. From these accounts, a fairly common pattern emerged, with some notable variations. Nearly all the victims cited three turning points after an initial "honeymoon" period; thus, I discerned four somewhat distinct phases of the relationship. The main variations were not whether these phases occurred, but how long they lasted, and how much they overlapped. The four phases of abuse are summarized in Box 2.1.

## Box 2.1 Summary of turning points in serious perpetrators' relationships with their victims

**First phase**
"Courtship" period ranges from one day to six months.
Couple begins to live together within three months on average.
Sex is usually daily or multiple times per day.
Perpetrator: Usually considerate, charming and romantic (though a quarter are abusive right away).
Victim: Loves partner, welcomes or acquiesces to his desire for frequent sex.

**Second phase**
Couple continues to have sex often.
Perpetrator: Commits first act of violence.
Victim: Complains about violence; some start to refuse sex.
Perpetrator: Apologizes for violence and promises it won't happen again.
Victim: Sees violence as an anomaly and accepts apology, resumes sex (either right away as part of perpetrator's "making up" or within one month).
Perpetrator: Feels that the status quo has been restored.

**Third phase**
Violence recurs and escalates.
Perpetrator: Continues to apologize but begins to ignore it and/or to blame her for it.
Victim: Becomes increasingly confused, unhappy, distrusting, and angry. Has thoughts of ending relationship. Resists partner in variety of ways that range from appeasement to defiance. Some victims separate for the first time, and/or seek help.
Perpetrator: Sensing victim unhappiness and resistance, further escalates his violence and seeks new ways to control her. If victim has separated this often includes monitoring, stalking, threats, rape, financial manipulation, and abuse or neglect of children.
Victim: Becomes more fearful, desperate, depressed and angry. Usually has turned to others for help and made one or more attempts to separate.
Perpetrator: Engages in forced, humiliating or rough sex. Begins to have affairs, and begins to compare victim to other women.
Victim: Most victims no longer refuse sex due to fear of consequences of refusal.
Perpetrator: Increasingly monitors victim, and during separations, stalks and threatens her.
Victim: Most who have left return to perpetrator due to fear or for financial reasons.

**Fourth phase**
Victim: Most are chronically unhappy, depressed, anxious and/or angry. Most make plans to leave or attempt to end relationship again.
Perpetrator: Further escalates his violence, threats and monitoring. Sex becomes increasingly violent and humiliating. He consistently blames victim for the violence and demands sex after violence.
Victim: Most no longer blame themselves or feel responsible for perpetrator's violence. Over half have ended the relationship.
Perpetrator: Monitors and stalks victim, demands sex as a way of reasserting control or claims of possession. When victim continues to resist or defy, he tries to kill her.

## First phase: Courtship

According to the victims, their courtship with the man who ultimately tried to kill them ranged from one day to six months, with a mean of 2.4 months. The courtship period includes the honeymoon period, which will be discussed later in this section. Courtship is defined as the time from when the couple first began to see each other to the time that they began to live together. For their part, 46% of the killers said that their courtship with the woman they killed was two months or less. For 31%, the courtship was one month or less, while for 12% it was one or two days. There were substantial differences between the men with shorter and longer courtships. Those with courtships of less than six months were older, with a mean age of 31 compared to 21.5 for those with courtships of over six months. Because they were older, the shorter courtship men had more life history. Part of that life history was more violence toward prior partners, more substance and drug abuse, more lost jobs, more problems with the law, and more failures in general. This may explain why these men have such short courtships; longer courtships would afford their partners more time to discover their past problems.

Another distinguishing feature of men with short courtships was the frequency of sex with their partners. Killers with short courtships were twice as likely to report having daily sex with their partners, with many of these saying that sex was multiple times a day. Sex also came much sooner in these relationships, most often during the first or second date. Though we did not ask all the victims of attempted homicide about how soon they had sex with their abusive partners, a similar pattern was revealed among the women who were asked. Overall, the victims of attempted homicide said that sex with their abusive partner came sooner and was more frequent than it had been with their prior or subsequent nonabusive partners. In retrospect, these women viewed early and frequent sex as warning signs that their partner might become an abuser. While these women said that they initially viewed sex as a sign of romantic affection, over time, most came to see it instead as an indicator of possessive control.

Though sex was soon and frequent, the majority of victims of attempted homicide reported that there had been a "honeymoon" phase to their relationship with their abuser. The honeymoon phase is the period of time before the first act of abuse. Notably, those with short courtships and earlier onset of sex reported that this was of shorter duration than those with longer courtships. For many women, the first act of abusive behavior did not come until after the onset of sexual relations, and by this they specified intercourse. Most victims said that prior to this, their partner was charming, thoughtful, and romantic, although there was a substantial subset of men (about one-quarter) who did not come across as such and were abusive from the outset. Again, these were overwhelmingly men who had abbreviated courtships with their partners.

For the men with shorter courtships, not only did their relationships begin sooner but they ended sooner as well. For the men with courtships of under six months, the average period of time from the beginning of the relationship to when they killed their partner was 4.25 years. This compared to 11.75 years for the killers with courtships of over six months.

## Second phase: Beginning of abuse

The first turning point, following the honeymoon period of the relationship, was when the man's abusive behavior first occurred. This was generally within the first year and soon after the couple began living together. The first incident was usually a mild to medium form of physical violence such as grabbing and shaking her, slapping her in the face, or pushing her against a wall. In no case was this sexual violence. In some cases, victims retrospectively recognized prior acts of nonviolent abusive behavior, such as criticisms or jealous accusations which they did not view as abusive at the time. In other cases, victims said that the physical violence was the first occurrence of abuse, which made it all the more surprising. Interestingly, the first incidents of violence often seemed to be triggered by jealous suspicions by the abuser.

> Annabel was seventeen and Wilberto was nineteen when they met through friends at a party. Annabel related that he came across as "fun-loving and gentle and shy." Two months after they started having a sexual relationship, Annabel and Wilberto attended a party with many mutual friends. At some point that evening, Annabel was shocked to see Wilberto fighting with another man. When she tried to intervene, Wilberto grabbed her by the shoulder and squeezed her arm, saying, "Why are you stopping me?" Only later at home did Wilberto apologize, telling Annabel that he'd had too much to drink.
>
> (Adams, 2007, p. 179)

Most victims felt shocked by the first act of violence since it was such a departure from their partner's behavior during the honeymoon period. Most victims expressed anger to their partners, and several threatened to end the relationship. Most stopped having sex with their partners. Almost without exception, the abuser apologized for this first act of violence and made the promise that it would not happen again. Significantly, all the victims who had stopped having sex agreed to resume it, in some cases upon his urging. In other cases, victims said they resumed sex since they welcomed the return of the tenderness and affection which had been present at the beginning of the relationship.

Ultimately, 90% of the victims of attempted murder said that their partners pressured them for sex on a daily or weekly basis, while 85% said that sex was forced. In comparison, 77% of the control group of women we interviewed reported that their partners had pressured them for sex, while 57% reported forced sex. It should be noted that this control group was drawn from women residing in an emergency shelter for abuse survivors and therefore was not necessarily reflective of abused women in general. However, one study that polled a presumably less extreme sample of women who had been physically abused – those seeking protective orders – found that 68% reported that they had been raped (McFarlane & Malecha, 2005). Another study that directly compared murder victims with a randomly identified control group of female abuse survivors found that the murder victims were four times more likely to have been raped by their abusive partner (Campbell, Webster, Koziol-McLain, & McFarlane, 2003).

## Third phase: Escalation of abuse, infidelity

The third phase was the continuation and gradual escalation of the man's abusive behavior, accompanied by a different kind of aftermath. The abuse now usually consisted of criticisms, jealous questions and accusations, and occasional or regular violence. For the most part, this came within months of the first act of violence, but in some cases occurred as long as a year later. During this phase, victims became increasingly confused, dissatisfied, and disillusioned about the relationship. They responded to the abuse in a variety of ways that ranged from fighting back to appeasing their partners. Some victims blamed themselves for their partner's jealous thoughts and began to limit their interactions with others. Cessation of sex, followed by "make up" sex within one hour to one week of an abusive incident was common. For the most part, the abusers were now less likely to apologize for their violence and began to ignore it. Several women talked about how confusing or "crazy making" this was. Edna said,

> He'd punch me in the face and when he came home later he'd be like, "Oh what's the matter, are you upset about something?". After a while, I began to imagine that maybe it was my imagination, except I still had the black eye.
>
> (Edna, personal communication, 2007)

Another common behavior by abusers during this period was infidelity. Some 75% of the women reported that their partners were having affairs. Revealingly, most of these women said that their partners took no pains to hide these affairs but in fact flaunted them. Of the 20 women, 6 said that partners would have sex with other women in their presence. Seven reported instances when the other woman would call their house to taunt them or to have extended conversations with their abusive partner. Some said their partners would openly compare them with the other woman (Adams, 2007):

As Lydia put it, "He told me I didn't know how to make him feel like a man."

Another victim, Anna, said, "He told me I was heavy in comparison to Sylvia (the other woman) . . . He would always comment about what a perfect body she has and, you know, how beautiful she is and this and that . . . Sometimes just out of the blue he'd say that . . . I was kind of shocked when he brought her over one day 'cause, you know, she wasn't that beautiful."

(p. 182)

Combined with abusers' growing tendency to blame their partners for their own abusive behavior, infidelity seemed to serve the purpose of putting women on the defensive. A number of women said that they felt insecure or inadequate as the result of their partner's involvement with other women.

Shelly, whose abuser lived part-time with another woman, said, "It made me feel so low . . . and I felt desperate really for his attention. Stupid me, he wasn't worth it, I can see that now but at the time I felt I was lucky to have him really."

(Adams, 2007, p. 182)

Some women worried that their partners would leave them for other women, not necessarily for fear of losing him but for fear of losing his financial support during a time when they had young children to raise. Three women said that their husbands threatened to "replace" them as mothers of their children with the other woman.

## Fourth phase: Further escalation and blaming the victim

Most victims of near-fatal assaults talked of a third turning point after the honeymoon period. During this phase there was a further step-up in the frequency and severity of violence. At the same time, the men were now consistently blaming their partners for the violence. For many women, this signified the point of no return: the realization that their partner's abusive behavior was not an anomaly but a normal and permanent feature of the relationship. Most of the women reported that their partners would now demand sex following an act of violence, and compliance with this was no longer negotiable. As Rose described it,

First I liked it when he was sweet-talking me and we'd end up back in bed together; but then it began to feel like rape.

(Rose, personal communication, 2007)

Another victim, Evie, discussed how her husband would treat her following an act of violence, "Oh he'd blame me, saying if I could act like a lady, he wouldn't have hurt me . . . He started demanding sex all the time. That was his way of making up but he would still be rough . . . that seemed to turn him on."

(Adams, 2007, p. 177)

Just over half of the victims said that their partners would regularly become violent during sex. Most of these women said that their partners appeared "excited," "aroused," or "turned on" by rough or violent sex. Infliction of pain during sex was a unilateral action on the part of the abusers. No victim said that her partner ever requested to be hit, slapped or bound in return. In many cases, sex was not just forced but humiliating. More than half reported insertion of objects in their vagina or rectum, and six women reported being urinated on. Six victims reported that their partner had demanded that they have sex with third-party adults.

One victim said, "He wanted me to do it [have sex with his friend] but then he would always throw it in my face afterward calling me a slut and a whore."

(Anonymous, personal communication, 2008)

Five victims reported that their abusers would sometimes insist on having sex in the presence of their children or other people. This not only served as a form of humiliation for the victim, but also as a form of potential blackmail. Three women said their husbands threatened to report to child welfare that they had sex in front of the children, resulting in the possible removal of the children.

Interestingly, the increasing severity and regularity of the violence, including the onset of sexual violence, helped most women to see that it was the man's problem and not something that she had "caused." It is important to note that most had children with their abusers by this time and because of this, said that they'd felt trapped in the relationship. The main entrapping factors that these women cited were economic dependency, fear of continued violence, and fear that he would attempt to take the children should she leave him. Some women said these fears were accompanied by growing depression and a sense of hopelessness about viable options.

While a few women said that they still loved their partners, a higher number said they no longer felt love or were ambivalent. Despite this, most said that within the first five years of the relationship, they began to have persistent thoughts about leaving. The women said that they began to feel chronically unhappy, angry and fearful. They engaged in a variety of passive and active resistance strategies. In terms of sexual relations, this ranged from angrily refusing to have sex to, as one woman put it, "just going through the motions."

In response to their partners' growing unhappiness and resistance, the perpetrators continued to escalate their abusive and coercive behaviors. These now included frequent jealous accusations and monitoring, as well as more severe forms of verbal and physical violence, including threats, sexual violence, rough sex, infidelity, and abuse or threats of abuse against the children. For the abuser, sex after violence seemed no longer a matter of "making up" for his violence but more about reinforcing the rules and reasserting his claims of ownership or possession. Five victims quoted their partners making ownership claims during sex that immediately followed violence. These included:

> "I don't care if you don't want to. You belong to me."
> "If I can't have you, nobody can."
> "I'm not playing games with you anymore."
> "I can do anything I want to you, whenever I want."
> "You think you're done with me bitch? You'll never be done with me. Got that?"
> "You are mine, remember that. I'll always have you."
>
> (Adams, 2007, p. 177)

Most of the women left their partners, temporarily or permanently, during this final phase. Abusers reacted to this with monitoring and stalking; terroristic threats; threats against the victim's friends and relatives; severe violence, including in public places; and sexual violence also in public places.

Sexual violence often continued after estrangement, appearing to be an attempt by perpetrators to reassert their claims of ownership over their victim.

> Dolores took her two-year-old son and fled her relationship with Elston to live with her best friend, Brenda. Two weeks later, Elston kicked open Brenda's front door. When Brenda tried to stop him, Elston punched her in the jaw. Then in the presence of his infant son, Elston threw Dolores on the floor and dragged her down two flights of stairs to his car. Elston then raped Dolores in his car that was parked on the street in front of Brenda's house with its driver's side door open, while loudly proclaiming, "You are mine, remember that. I'll always have you."
>
> (Adams, 2007, p. 249)

In a number of instances, the final near-fatal assault committed by the abuser was triggered by the victim's refusal to have sex (Adams, 2007):

> Annabel reported that Wilberto attempted to kill her after she refused to have sex. Enraged at her defiance, Wilberto severely beat her with his fists and then began hitting her over the head with a metal fan. He stopped only after he felt her neck for a pulse and was apparently convinced that she had died.
>
> (p. 179)

In some cases, the final act of attempted homicide included rape. One victim reported that following her estrangement from her partner, he abducted her into his car and raped her while holding a gun to her head.

(p. 249)

Several of the killers reported that rape immediately preceded their killing their partner. In the case of John, who was 29 when he killed his wife Debra, the fatal encounter occurred after their separation. Debra let John come over to her parents' house to see their small daughters, with the proviso that her brother be there. After the brother and the little girls were in bed,

> . . . at John's insistence they watched a sexually provocative video named Body Heat. During this time, John served Debra two mixed drinks, knowing from past experience that alcohol would make her sleepy. He then coerced Debra to have sex. When Debra fell asleep, John took the two girls out of bed and put them in his car. He then went back in the house, and while Debra lay asleep, plunged a large hunting knife into her neck and then bludgeoned her over the head with a baseball bat. He then drove the girls around Cape Cod for several hours before turning himself in to the police. During my interview with him six years later, John explained his decision to have sex with Debra before killing her since, "It was a way of preserving us as a couple forever." He added that he also wanted Debra's (presumed) new boyfriend to know that "I was the last to have her" (Adams, 2007, p. 167).
>
> Another killer, Harold, lured his estranged partner, Jenaya, to stay at a hotel with him after suspecting that she had been with another man. After having sex with her, Harold shot her in the head before shooting himself in the stomach. Harold survived the shooting, telling me 7 years later that Jenaya "could have saved herself if she just admitted it (the presumed affair)."
>
> (Adams, 2007, p. 169)

## Understanding sexual assault by lethal abusers

When one examines how and when sexual assaults occur in the context of the relationship, these acts appear to be an integral element of the serious abuser's repertoire of possessive control tactics. Early sex in their relationships seems to signify his beginning claims of exclusive ownership, or at least the presumption of exclusive sexual access. Frequent sex serves both as a replacement for emotional intimacy and as a form of camouflage for the early stages of possessive control. "Make-up" sex serves to restore the status quo and to smooth over tensions after incidents of abuse. For some victims, sex after violence was welcomed as a sign of tenderness and interest, and as a temporary compensation for the hurt she had suffered from his abuse, and, in some cases, as a hope that things could get better. Over time, sex after violence became more a means of temporarily pacifying the abuser and of forestalling future abuse.

For the abuser, rough, painful, and humiliating sex serves to diminish his partner's will by reinforcing the message that he can do whatever he wishes. Many of the victims we interviewed said that sexual violence and humiliation made them feel depressed, ashamed, hopeless and self-loathing. For the abuser, sexual humiliation of the victim often helps to further his social isolation of his partner by creating experiences that she is loath to disclose to others who might otherwise be sources of support. Sexual humiliation also seems to be a central element in the abuser's objectification of his partner as subhuman "property." Such debasement only cements his perception of her as an object to be used as he wishes.

> As one abuser I counseled once noted, "Once I reduced her to rubble, once I started treating her like a piece of furniture, her feelings didn't really matter . . . and I stopped thinking of her as a real person."
> (Anonymous, personal communication, 2004)

> Another man reflected, "I pressured her to do whatever sick things I wanted, have sex whenever and however I wanted it, have sex with me and other women, and then she was a slut and a whore in my eyes."
> (Anonymous, personal communication, 2008)

More than any other single element of domestic abuse, sexual coercion and violence appear to be the sine qua non tactic of the abuser's attempts to gain and maintain possessive control over his partner. Early on in the relationship, he relies on sexual coercion, and sometimes infidelity, to diminish his partner's sense of will and autonomy and to impose his sexual prerogative. Later, he relies on sexual humiliation to devalue his partner to the point where she becomes a more palatable or justifiable target of his violence. Sexual violence reinforces this objectification and further serves as a way for the abuser to reassert possessive control in response to his partner's resistance.

Sexual violence is a risk factor to intimate partner homicide because it reveals the abuser's willingness to completely ignore his partner's wishes. At the same time, it demonstrates his attempts to repossess or to punish her when she attempts to end the relationship. Possessive sexual violence reveals a motive for murder: a desire on the abuser's part to punish his partner for her defiance, and for her presumed intentions to replace him with someone else.

## References

Adams, D. (2007). *Why do they kill? Men who murder their intimate partners.* Nashville, TN: Vanderbilt University Press.

Adams, D., & Cayouette, S. (2002). Emerge: A group model for abusers. In E. Aldarondo & F. Mederos (Eds.), *Programs for men who batter: Intervention and prevention strategies in a diverse society*. New York, NY: Civic Research.

Campbell, J.D., Webster, J., Koziol-McLain, C., & McFarlane, C. (2003). Risk factors for intimate partner homicide. *American Journal of Public Health, 93*, 1089–1097.

Dobash, R.E., & Dobash, R.P. (1979). *Violence against wives: A case against the patriarchy*. New York, NY: Free Press.

Dobash, R.E., & Dobash, R.P. (2015). *When men murder women*. Oxford, UK: Oxford University Press.

Gondolf, E. (2002). *Batterer intervention systems: Issues, outcomes and recommendations*.Thousand Oaks, CA: Sage.

McFarlane, J., & Malecha, A. (2005). Sexual assaults among intimates: Frequency, consequences and treatment. National Institute of Justice. Retrieved from: www.ncjrs.gov/pdffiles/nij/grants/211678.pdf.

# Chapter 3

# Children's exposure to intimate partner sexual violence

*Kathryn Ford*

Sexual violence that occurs in the context of intimate partner relationships is often misunderstood or overshadowed by physical abuse, and cases involving both domestic violence and sexual assault present myriad barriers to effective therapeutic and criminal justice responses. In addition, interventions and research into children's exposure to domestic violence have focused almost solely on physical violence, despite the fact that children can and do witness sexual assaults against adults in their homes. Addressing this issue is critical to any effort to support the safety and well-being of victimized parents and their children, to provide children with clinical support around severely traumatic experiences, and to hold offenders accountable for the full extent and impact of their violent and abusive behavior.

In this chapter, I provide statistics and case examples that illustrate many of the dynamics and effects of children's exposure to intimate partner sexual violence (IPSV). I also offer some ideas for research priorities and recommended practices for clinical intervention and justice system response.

## Prevalence of intimate partner sexual violence

IPSV is a rarely discussed but unfortunately common form of violent victimization that often co-occurs with other types of intimate partner violence. Numerous studies indicate that between 45% and 75% of women who are physically abused by an intimate partner have been sexually assaulted by their partner as well (Campbell et al., 1997; McCloskey et al., 2002). The trauma to the adult victim is often severe, involving emotional and physical effects that are equal to or greater in severity than the symptoms experienced by individuals who are sexually assaulted by other types of perpetrators, or who are physically but not sexually abused by their partner (Campbell & Soeken, 1999; Cole et al., 2005). Some of this differential impact may be accounted for by the unique dynamics of IPSV, such as the severe sense of betrayal felt by the victim, reluctance to label the incidents as sexual violence, and the frequently chronic nature of intimate partner sexual assault. It is also critical to note that sexual assault in an intimate relationship is statistically correlated with more severe and frequent physical violence by the abusive partner, more severe threats and psychological abuse, increased risk of abuse during pregnancy, more severe stalking, and domestic violence homicide perpetration and victimization (Campbell et al., 2003; Coker et al., 2000; Martin et al., 2004).

## Children's exposure to sexual violence in the home

Although there is increasing research being conducted on the prevalence and dynamics of sexual assault in intimate relationships, one of the most neglected areas of inquiry is how often children are exposed to such incidents and how they are affected. In the only published study to document the frequency of children's exposure, Campbell and Alford (1989) conducted research interviews with 115 women residing in a domestic violence shelter, all of whom had been raped by their male partner. Nearly 18% reported that their children had witnessed at least one incident of sexual assault and 5.2% reported that their partner had involved the children in a forced sex act. Clearly, these statistics do not include children's exposure to sexual violence of which the victimized parent is unaware, such as a child overhearing an incident from another room or walking in as an assault is being perpetrated.

Despite the dearth of formal research in this area, anecdotal evidence and clinical experience indicate that there are many ways children are involved in and affected by their exposure to sexual violence. These include being visual or hearing witnesses, attempting to verbally or physically intervene during an assault, and being forced to participate in the sexual assault of a parent. The abusive adult may intentionally sexually assault the adult victim in the presence of children; maintain poor sexual boundaries with children, including discussing the adult sexual relationship with them; use sexually degrading language toward their partner in front of the children; or even force their partner to have sexual contact with a child. Abusers may also use the children to sexually coerce their partner – for example, by threatening to sexually abuse the children, prevent parent–child contact, or withhold child support or other resources if she doesn't comply.

## Impact of IPSV on children

For children, witnessing the rape of a parent is an experience distressing enough to trigger the development of posttraumatic stress disorder (Pynoos & Nader, 1988). In addition, IPSV is associated with more severe depression, anxiety, and behavior problems in children, as compared to those whose mothers have been physically, but not sexually, abused (McFarlane & Malecha, 2005; Symes et al., 2014). IPSV is also statistically correlated with impairment of the bond between mother and child, likely due to the effects of the sexual violence on the mother's mental health and well-being (Goncalves Boeckel, Wagner, & Grassi-Oliveira, 2015).

As a result of their exposure to sexual violence, children may also internalize distorted and unhealthy messages about gender, sexuality, and sexual consent, such as:

*   sexuality, coercion and violence are inextricably intertwined;
*   men have a right to sex at any time and women are obligated to provide it;
*   sexuality is not something to be enjoyed and shared, but to be feared;
*   sexual aggression is normal and justifiable;
*   sexuality can be used to control, degrade, and humiliate one's partner; and
*   if one wants sex, one should take it without regard for the wishes of one's partner.

Furthermore, sexual violence in the adult relationship is associated with the abuser threatening violence toward the children and perpetrating direct emotional and/or physical child abuse (McFarlane & Malecha, 2005; McFarlane et al., 2005). Domestic violence is also a known risk factor for child sexual abuse – one study found that men who abuse their adult partners are 6.5 times more likely to sexually abuse their children, and identified intimate partner violence as one of only four statistically significant predictors of intrafamilial child sexual abuse (Paveza, 1988). However, it's unknown at this time whether perpetration of sexual violence toward one's partner indicates an even greater level of risk of perpetrating child sexual abuse.

Lastly, IPSV increases the likelihood of the victim experiencing reproductive health difficulties that are related to children's health and well-being, such as forced or prohibited abortion, unwanted or poorly spaced pregnancies, infertility, miscarriage, stillbirth, and sexually transmitted infection during pregnancy (Bennice & Resick, 2003; McFarlane et al., 2005).

## Legal history

Several legal cases of note provide further documentation of children's exposure to sexual violence. Oregon v. Rideout, 108, 866 Circuit Court, County of Marion, Oregon (1978) was the first nationally publicized case of marital rape. It was also the first prosecution for an incident that occurred while the parties were still living together. Mr. Rideout was charged with beating and raping his wife in front of their two-year-old daughter but was eventually acquitted. In contrast, in People v. Liberta, 64 N.Y.2d 152 (1984), the assault occurred post-separation while an Order of Protection was in effect. The defendant was convicted of repeatedly raping and sodomizing his estranged wife in a hotel room in front of their young son, after she had gone there seeking to exchange the child for visitation. Lastly, in People v. Parr, 548 N.Y.S.2d 121; 155 A.D.2d 945 (1989), the defendant was convicted of Endangering the Welfare of a

Child, among other crimes, for raping and sodomizing a woman in the presence of her five-year-old son. The New York State Court of Appeals ruled that this was an appropriate use of the Endangering statute due to the severe psychological trauma to the child.

## Case examples

The following cases from our clinical practice illustrate the ways children are exposed and respond to IPSV, the impact of this experience on their emotional well-being, and some of the impediments to successfully prosecuting these cases and providing support to child and adult victims. These cases also provide a glimpse of the behavior of IPSV perpetrators with regard to the children in their households, which is an important consideration in designing appropriate interventions for perpetrators.

## Case example I

Emily is an eight-year-old girl. For two years, she was exposed to increasingly violent emotional and physical abuse directed toward her mother, Ms. R., by the mother's boyfriend, Mr. A. One evening, Mr. A. became enraged that Ms. R. did not have dinner ready on time and threw a pork chop at her face. After punching and kicking her several times, Mr. A. ripped off Ms. R.'s clothes and raped her in the living room, in Emily's presence. Upon hearing her mother's cries for help, Emily began screaming at Mr. A. to stop, striking him repeatedly on the head and back with a plastic baseball bat. Within hours of the incident, Ms. R. called the police, and Mr. A. was arrested and charged with rape in the first degree and several counts of physical assault.

During her brief time in therapy, Emily reported pervasive feelings of anxiety and fear, described seeing herself in the caretaking role in relation to her mother, and drew a picture of herself jumping head-first off a mountain and bleeding from a head injury. A few months later, after the highest charge had been reduced to attempted rape in the second degree, the criminal case went to trial. As the only witness to the incident, Emily was called to testify against Mr. A., who was sitting in the courtroom before her. A victim advocate prepared Emily for her testimony and court experience and accompanied her to court. However, Emily met only briefly with the prosecutor, who had never worked with a child witness and had limited expertise in the prosecution of sexual violence. As a result, Emily and the prosecutor had difficulty communicating while Emily was on the witness stand, and she was unable to describe what she had experienced in a clear and detailed manner. The jury returned a sole conviction for misdemeanor physical assault, acquitting Mr. A. of all sexual assault charges, and Mr. A. was sentenced to five months in jail with credit for time served.

## Case example 2

Aleya is a 14-year-old girl. Her stepfather, Mr. B., abused alcohol and was emotionally, physically, and sexually abusive to Aleya's mother, Ms. B. Mr. B. would often make sexually degrading comments to Ms. B. in front of Aleya and her 7-year-old brother, and would watch pornography in the living room when the children were present despite Ms. B.'s pleas that he refrain until the children had gone to sleep. Mr. B. also raped and sexually coerced Ms. B. on a regular basis.

On one occasion, Mr. B. came home drunk in the middle of the night. Ms. B. and the children, who had fallen asleep together on the living room couch, woke up to the sound of Mr. B. loudly demanding that his wife give him sex. Ms. B. cried that she would not have sex with him in front of the children, and Mr. B. threatened to kill her if she didn't take her clothing off. When Ms. B. continued to refuse, Mr. B. began threatening her with a knife and demanded that Aleya go into the bathroom and wait for him. Aleya, concerned for her mother's life, followed his instructions. When Mr. B. arrived in the bathroom, he orally raped Aleya by threatening to kill her mother if she did not comply. He told Aleya that it was her mother's refusal to fulfill his sexual needs that was causing him to turn to her.

While Mr. B. was raping Aleya in the bathroom, Ms. B. called the police. Mr. B. was arrested and charged with menacing, endangering the welfare of a child, and sodomy in the first degree. Ms. B. and Aleya were referred for therapy by the District Attorney's Office, at which point Aleya shared that she was having thoughts of suicide, frequently felt sad, was having nightmares, and was afraid that Mr. B. would return to the home. (This case was provided by Amy Pumo, LCSW, Director of the Center for Court Innovation's Bronx Child and Adolescent Witness Support Program.)

## Case example 3

Ethan is a 7-year-old boy. His father, Mr. L., severely abused his mother, Ms. P., over many years, which included sex trafficking, frequent rapes and beatings, tying her up for hours at a time, burning her with hot liquid, and stalking. Mr. L. deliberately humiliated Ms. P. in many ways, including by laughingly grabbing and hitting her breasts and buttocks, and calling her sexually degrading names in front of Ethan. Mr. L. also physically abused Ethan and did not maintain appropriate boundaries with him.

When Ethan began therapy, he had severe symptoms of posttraumatic stress disorder, significant behavioral problems at school and at home, and academic and developmental delays due to his lifelong exposure to domestic violence. The behavioral concerns included acting disrespectfully toward women and girls, including his teachers, masturbating in front of Ms. P., hitting Ms. P., and grabbing Ms. P.'s breasts and laughing, as he had seen his father do. His relationship with Ms. P. had also been damaged by the abuse – Ethan did not respect his mother or see her as a source of protection and support.

Once Ms. P. and Ethan were able to relocate to a safe place away from Mr. L., Ethan's therapy focused on assisting him with managing his trauma symptoms, providing psychoeducation about healthy and abusive relationships, and strengthening his relationship with his mother, including helping her to understand his behaviors and how they related to the trauma he experienced, coaching her in how to set appropriate boundaries with him and respond effectively when he acted hurtfully, and supporting her in asserting an active parenting role for the first time.

## Best practices for intervention

Children's exposure to intimate partner sexual violence is a very new area for both practice and research. However, based on clinical experience and the limited research available, the following practices are recommended:

- Screen all victims of intimate partner violence for sexual abuse in their relationships, using behavioral descriptions rather than legal terms. (For example, a provider might say: "Many of the clients I work with who've been hurt physically by their partner have also been hurt in a sexual way. Has your partner ever forced you to do something sexual against your will or without your permission?")
- Prior to inquiring about children's potential exposure to and involvement in sexual violence, advise clients about any limits to confidentiality that are inherent to your professional role, such as mandated reporting of child abuse and neglect.
- If sexual violence is disclosed by a parent, ask if children have witnessed or been involved directly in the sexual violence, and, if so, how the children responded.
- In addition, assess for threats to abuse the children, actual emotional, physical and/or sexual abuse of children, and risk factors for lethality and escalation of violence.

Other recommendations include:

- Facilitate adult victims' access to reproductive health care services, and incorporate sexual violence and birth-control concerns into safety planning.
- Specifically address sexual violence experiences, healthy boundaries, and sexual decision-making as part of therapeutic interventions with exposed children.
- Where appropriate, prosecute abusers for exposing children to sexual violence and/or involving them in sexually violent acts.

- Provide training on skills for interviewing children and working with child witnesses to all law enforcement officers and prosecutors who work with domestic violence and/or sexual assault cases.
- In all contexts, including decision-making regarding child custody and visitation, consider intimate partner sexual violence as an indicator of increased risk of harm to children and adult victims both pre- and post-separation.
- Evaluate and collect data on all interventions and outcomes, as a way of contributing to the research literature and helping to identify and inform the development of safe and effective practices.

## Research questions and priorities

As noted previously, very little research has been conducted on children's exposure to intimate partner sexual violence. As a result, there are numerous questions and issues that are ripe for research and data collection, the answers to which would provide important guidance to criminal justice personnel and service providers. These include:

- How prevalent is children's exposure to intimate partner sexual violence, in community and clinical samples?
- In what ways are the effects of children's exposure to sexual violence similar to and different from exposure to physical violence and other types of abuse?
- Are children exposed to sexual violence more likely to perpetrate sexual violence as teens or adults and/or to be victimized by a partner? If so, what are the mechanisms of the intergenerational transmission of sexual violence?
- In what ways do abused mothers protect their children from exposure to sexual violence or respond when such exposure does occur?
- Are men who use sexual violence against their adult partners more likely to perpetrate child sexual abuse than men who solely perpetrate physical violence?
- What methods of screening and assessment, with both children and victimized parents, are most effective?
- How can therapeutic interventions with children, in individual and group settings, sensitively and effectively address exposure to sexual violence?
- How does the presence of a child witness influence the criminal justice response to reported incidents of intimate partner sexual violence?
- How can children best be supported when they are called to testify about the rape of a parent?
- In what ways can the criminal justice system improve its response to children who are exposed to sexual violence?

## Conclusion

Victim service providers and legal system personnel have made significant strides over the past 20 years in understanding and responding to children's experiences of domestic violence. However, exposure to the sexual abuse of a parent has been a seriously neglected issue, despite its potentially severe traumatic impact on children and association with greater risk to the safety and well-being of children and adult victims. It is essential that as practitioners and researchers we move beyond our emotional discomfort with this difficult subject to find answers to pressing questions, provide much needed supportive intervention to those affected, and hold abusers accountable for the physical and psychological harm they inflict.

## References

Bennice, J.A., & Resick, R.A. (2003). Marital rape: History, research, and practice. *Trauma, Violence, & Abuse, 4*(3), 228–246.

Campbell, J.C., & Alford, R. (1989). The dark consequences of marital rape. *American Journal of Nursing, 89*, 946–949.

Campbell, J.C., & Soeken, K.L. (1999). Forced sex and intimate partner violence: Effects on women's risk and women's health. *Violence Against Women, 5*(9), 1017–1035.

Campbell, J.C., Kub, J., Belknap, R., & Templin, T.N. (1997). Predictors of depression in battered women. *Violence Against Women, 3*(3), 271–293.

Campbell, J.C., Webster, D., Koziol-McLain, J., Block, C.R., Campbell, D., Curry, M., Gary, F., McFarlane, J., Sachs, C., Sharps, P., Ulrich, Y., & Wilt, S.A. (2003). Assessing risk factors for intimate partner homicide. *National Institutes of Justice Journal, 250*, 14–19.

Coker, A.L., Hall Smith, P., McKeown, R.E., & King, M.J. (2000). Frequency and correlates of intimate partner violence by type: Physical, sexual, and psychological battering. *American Journal of Public Health, 90*(4), 553–559.

Cole, J., Logan, T., & Shannon, L. (2005). Intimate sexual victimization among women with protective orders: Types and associations of physical and mental health problems. *Violence and Victims, 20*(6), 695–715.

Goncalves Boeckel, M., Wagner, A., & Grassi-Oliveira, R. (2015). The effects of intimate partner violence exposure on the maternal bond and PTSD symptoms of children. *Journal of Interpersonal Violence, 1–16.*

McCloskey, L.A., Treviso, M., Scionti, T., & dal Pozzo, G. (2002). A comparative study of battered women and their children in Italy and the United States. *Journal of Family Violence, 17*(1), 53–74.

McFarlane, J. & Malecha, A. (2005). *Sexual assault among intimates: Frequency, consequences & treatments.* Rockville, MD: National Criminal Justice Reference Service.

McFarlane, J., Malecha, A., Watson, K., Gist, J., Batten, E., Hall, I. & Smith, S. (2005). Intimate partner sexual assault against women: Frequency, health consequences, and treatment outcomes. *Obstetrics & Gynecology, 105*(1), 99–108.

Martin, S.L., Harris-Britt, A., Li, Y., Moracco, K.E., Kupper, L.L., & Campbell, J.C. (2004). Changes in intimate partner violence during pregnancy. *Journal of Family Violence, 19*(4), 201–210.

Paveza, G.J. (1988). Risk factors in father–daughter child sexual abuse: A case-control study. *Journal of Interpersonal Violence, 3*(3), 290–306.

Pynoos, R.S., & Nader, K. (1988). Children who witness the sexual assaults of their mothers. *Journal of the American Academy of Child and Adolescent Psychiatry, 27*, 567–572.

Symes, L., Maddoux, J., McFarlane, J., Nava, A., & Gilroy, H. (2014). Physical and sexual intimate partner violence, women's health and children's behavioural functioning: Entry analysis of a seven-year prospective study. *Journal of Clinical Nursing, 23*(19–20), 2909–2918.

# Who are the perpetrators of intimate partner sexual violence?

# Chapter 4

# The mindset of intimate partner sexual violence perpetrators

## Motivations and myths

*Patricia Easteal and Louise McOrmond-Plummer*

In this chapter we look at intimate partner sexual violence (IPSV) perpetrators' motivations and the myths that they may subscribe to in order to justify their sexual violence and avoid taking responsibility. By exploring the psychological and social factors that contribute to the mindset of men who rape, we aim to reduce victim-blaming and increase the understanding that is required to underpin prevention. Our aim in the chapter is also to challenge myths about who are "real" rapists.

## Motivation

First, while many people do not consider the partner rapist to be a "real" rapist in the same sense as a stranger rapist, as we see in the table below, the motivations for rape are remarkably similar whether the victim is a stranger or a partner.

Through some examples reported by survivors, we now look more closely at motives of rapists, and partner rapists in particular. Please bear in mind also that just because a perpetrator of IPSV may be motivated by anger on some occasions, for example, that does not mean this is always his motivation. Motivations may change due to the circumstances. For example, a man who forces his partner into sexual activity without additional physical violence with the aim of establishing control over her, may, at another time, beat her severely in the course of a rape because the aim is punishment (Easteal & McOrmond-Plummer, 2006).

## Power/control

IPSV is often a manifestation of intimate coercion (Leone, Johnson, & Cohan, 2007). A subtext is evident in this type of family violence: domination, intimidation, and control (Kelly & Johnson, 2008). It is far easier to exert power over someone who has been emotionally degraded and feels worthless. Sexual assault is one means the offender may use to disempower and humiliate. The ability to subjugate a woman with his penis may give a man a sense of mastery

Table 4.1 Reasons given for rape

| Reasons given for rape | The partners | The strangers |
|---|---|---|
| **Power** | "It gave me a certain feeling of power over her because I knew she found it unpleasurable. It was one of the only times I could best her" (Finkelhor & Yllo, 1985, p. 65). | "At that time, it gave me a sense of power. A sense of accomplishing something that I felt I didn't have the ability to get" (Russell, 1975, p. 244). |
| **Anger/retaliation** | "I guess I was angry at her. It was a way of getting even" (Finkelhor & Yllo, 1985, p. 80). | "I met a girl at a party . . . she irritated me . . . I took her home to her apartment and I raped her" (Russell, 1975, p. 253). |
| **Insecurity/sense of inadequacy** | "She was a stronger person than I was in many ways, and I had an inferiority complex about it" (Finkelhor & Yllo, 1985, p. 79). | "I raped about four chicks . . . they all had a certain self-assurance . . . it used to be threatening to me" (Russell, 1975, p. 252). |
| **Sexually aroused by causing pain/fear** | "I had the best erection I'd had in years. It was very stimulating. I walked around with a smile on my face for three days. You could say, I suppose, that I raped her" (Finkelhor & Yllo, 1985, p. 66). | "*Interviewer:* Did her fear turn you on?<br>*Rapist:* Yes.<br>*Interviewer:* How did you feel about her being hurt?<br>*Rapist:* That was exciting"<br>(Russell, 1975, p. 246). |
| **Preference for coercive sex over consensual sex** | "I get this satisfaction from a feeling of some dominance – a man over woman thing" (Finkelhor & Yllo, 1985, p. 81). | "Making a girl wouldn't do it . . . It was the unattainable I wanted" (Russell, 1975, p. 245). |
| **Sense of entitlement** | "I have a right to this" (Finkelhor & Yllo, 1985, p. 76). | "You want this, and you don't see why you can't have it so you take it" (Russell, 1975, p. 245). |

Source: Easteal & McOrmond-Plummer, 2006, p. 66. Reproduced with permission of Hybrid

over feelings of inadequacy and weakness; it reaffirms his masculinity (Groth & Birnbaum, 1979).

The rapist motivated by power, particularly in the context of IPSV, may negate consent with emotional coercion:

> The best way I can describe it is that there was an unspoken threat that if I didn't have sex with him he would emotionally abuse me. He would throw a tantrum if I said no, guilt trip me. Ignore me, reject me, and because he had convinced me that I was in love with him and couldn't live without him these things hurt me a lot so in a way, I submitted to sex because it was the only way to avoid emotional/mental pain.
>
> (Easteal & McOrmond-Plummer, 2006, p. 67)

Verbal badgering is not a legitimate request for sex that permits the victim to say no without unpleasant consequences – the perpetrator's intention is "Give me sex or I'll take it."

If verbal coercion is unsuccessful, physical force is likely to be used (Englander, 2003). The rapist driven by the need for power uses whatever force may be necessary to achieve sexual intercourse. He may sometimes use slapping or weapons to show his victim he means "business"; yet, according to Groth & Birnbaum (1979), sexual possession of the woman to satisfy his need for power is his main aim, rather than hurting her physically.

Because rape motivated by power may lack the physical violence of more stereotypical "violent" rape, victims are often confused and angry with themselves, believing that they could have done more to stop it. The perpetrator, both nonverbally and through speech, may try to make the victim feel complicit:

> I told him no, that I didn't want to do it – he kept going, when I kept saying no he stopped briefly, he started abusing me (verbally) telling me that it was all my fault and that I kept leading him on.
>
> (Easteal & McOrmond-Plummer, 2006, p. 67)

The rapist who is motivated primarily by a need for power (labeled as the "power rapist" in Groth's 1979 typology) may not see any harm in his actions, or he has no empathy or regard for the victim's feelings: "During the worst incident I did cry and he was aware of this, despite the fact that I was doing my best to conceal my tears. He did not stop" (Easteal & McOrmond Plummer, 2006, p. 68).

Indeed, as opposed to seeing his behavior from the victim's point of view, the rapist motivated by power often needs to convince himself that his victim has enjoyed his attention: "He would say that I wanted it; he would say that I wouldn't be here if I didn't want it" (Easteal & McOrmond-Plummer, 2006, p. 106). With IPSV, rape might occur as a means of glossing over an argument or other types of violence that he has inflicted:

And after the physical pain, always came the demands for intimacy. I hated it. I hated it all. In my experience it is used to re-affirm their "love" of the victim and that "now everything is back to normal." As if nothing has happened. As if the sexual act itself wipes out all unpleasantness.

(Easteal & McOrmond Plummer, 2006, p. 68)

As with other expressions of intimate terrorism, when the perpetrator's control of his partner is challenged by her leaving the relationship, he may respond with violence. Rape might be an act of "repossession" (Russell, 1990, p.153). Therefore, not surprisingly, it is not unusual for sexual assaults to take place or even to begin following separation (DeKeseredy, 2014).

Sexual assault is still continuing. He is always kissing me. Feeling my breasts, in between my legs – "just as friends." He has had sex with me twice in 4 weeks, even though I have told him I don't want to. He has stayed at my house the past 3 nights and although I have managed to stop him having sex, he always tries. Again, according to him, this is just being good friends. I have told him that I feel as though he is still trying to control me.

(Easteal & McOrmond Plummer, 2006, p. 68)

## Anger/punishment

Much rape contains elements of anger, and in rape largely fueled by anger there are power and control issues too. Anger, though, may be the primary motivator:

But I felt so dirty all the time. I spent hours in the shower, even when the water was running freezing, even when there was no more soap, I used cleaning products. My time in the shower angered him. Sometimes he was so angry that he had sex with me when I got out. He demanded I leave the bathroom door unlocked, as he felt he should be able to look at me any time he wanted.

(Easteal & McOrmond Plummer, 2006, p. 69)

The rapist mainly motivated by anger commonly uses rape to punish and humiliate a woman (Holmes & Holmes, 2002). Because retribution is the primary aim, rape may include particularly humiliating acts such as ejaculating on the victim's face or in her hair (Shapcott, 1988). These rapes thus commonly include forced oral and anal sex as the perpetrator perceives that his victim will find them painful and degrading (Easteal & McOrmond-Plummer, 2006).

He said, "I am going to come on your face, I can't wait to come on your face." I was silent for a bit, and he repeated himself . . . "I can't wait to come all over your fucking face." . . . I turned around and soon, in that deep voice he said, "I am going to fuck you up the ass. Yeah, fuck you right up the ass. You're going to like it, bitch"

(Easteal & McOrmond Plummer, 2006, p. 114)

When anger is at the core of the act, the rapist is likely to use other physical violence such as slapping or biting (Groth & Birnhaum, 1979): "He was sometimes very violent during sex. He would hit, pinch, or beat me during or prior to intercourse, or for refusing to submit" (Easteal & McOrmond Plummer, 2006, p. 69).

Unlike the rapist who is motivated primarily by power who forces sex on his partner after beating her in order to manipulate her feelings, for the partner who is primarily motivated by anger, the beating is *part* of the rape: "He often wanted sex after beating me. The battering seemed part punishment and part foreplay" (Easteal & McOrmond Plummer, 2006, p. 69).

Eventually he couldn't have sex with me unless he hurt me first. He would explode, scream and yell and break things, batter my heart and my body and then want to make love to make it all better. Sex itself was not violent just all that led up to it.

(Easteal & McOrmond Plummer, 2006, p. 28)

I was woken late at night or early hours of the morning and slapped across the face whilst I was in a half-dazed state because I refused his demands and asked not to be woken.

One time he positioned himself behind me and held my chin, head and shoulders. He proceeded to pull my head to the side as if to break my neck. He then pushed me to the ground and straddled me, he placed his knees on my arms pinning them to the floor, and with one hand he held his hand over my nose and mouth to stop me screaming in pain and horror. He had his other hand around my throat, strangling me, whilst he told me that he wished I were dead.

(Easteal & McOrmond Plummer, 2006, p. 69)

In Shapcott's (1988) typology, in anger rape, the victim may be coerced into playing a role in the degradation.

I was forced to take my clothes off while he sat in a chair in front of me with a knife in his hand. He wanted me to take my clothes off slowly and when he felt that it wasn't slow enough he would get up and hit me again and tell me that I better "start fucking listening."

(Easteal & McOrmond Plummer 2006, p. 70)

In addition, men who rape in anger may show a tendency to "snap" suddenly, changing from relatively pleasant to angry and violent (Groth & Birnbaum, 1979).

Just when I thought I could predict him, he would react to something in a way completely apart from what I expected . . . He had been wonderful that night – sweet and charming and why I started dating him in the first place. Then, halfway into the movie, he became moody and said it was time to go. He was angry at me and hit me and raped me that night.

(Easteal & McOrmond Plummer, 2006, p. 70)

Anger rapists may act tough and overtly appear very "macho." However, their self-image is likely to be quite fragile. Perhaps due to this inner sense of fragility, the anger rapist may release rage onto women he sees as having belittled or bested him in some way. Sex is his weapon of contempt. He uses it to "make hate" to his victim (Shapcott, 1988, p. 39): "Looking back, I can see that when he felt inferior or upset was when he tended to be more abusive towards me (like when he would fail an exam or get a speeding ticket)" (Easteal & McOrmond Plummer, 2006, p. 71).

Accordingly, threat to his sense of sexual ownership may be a precursor to rape. Rape may be punishment for her behavior:

The thing I will never forget is when we went to watch Robbie Williams in concert . . . When we got home, he flew into one of his rages, screaming that I fancied Robbie more than him . . . accusing me of wanting to do this . . . and he went down on me, biting my vagina with such force that he lifted my bottom half off the bed with his teeth.

(Easteal & McOrmond Plummer, 2006, p. 71)

It may be retribution for daring to end the relationship:

I was raped vaginally, anally and was also forced to perform oral sex. He was armed with a knife that was held against me at various times through-out the rape. I was beaten very badly with a closed fist as well as an open hand. I was also held tightly around my throat, which was restricting my ability to breathe. I was also knocked into a filing cabinet which caused bleeding. He was also banging my head against the filing cabinet and the floor. I bled quite a bit from being raped anally. I was left quite bruised and bloody from the rape and the beating.

(Easteal & McOrmond Plummer, 2006, p. 72)

## Sadism

Although rape motivated primarily by anger often does contain sadistic acts, the difference between anger rape and sadistic rape is that where the anger rapist hurts his victim to punish her, the sadistic rapist causes her pain and terror in order to arouse *himself* (Groth & Birnbaum, 1979). Despite the apparent rarity of sadistically motivated rape, it is clear that it does happen within the IPSV context (Frances & Wollert, 2012).

The rapist finds the intentional maltreatment of his victim intensely gratifying, and takes pleasure in her torment, anguish, distress, helplessness, and suffering. The assault usually involves bondage and torture, and frequently has a bizarre or ritualistic quality to it with the insertion of objects into the victim, together with extra tortures such as biting, burning, or cutting her body (Hucker, 1997).

> He bit and pinched my breasts and told me to roll over. When I resisted he acted as though he was going to put the blade into me and so I rolled onto my stomach. He then proceeded to penetrate me anally, punching me in the back, calling me a whore and a little cry-baby. I tried to get up, but he would punch me right in the center of my back, it was taking my breath away. He then rolled me over and went down on me, biting the inside of my thighs and squeezing my breasts so hard, he left bruises . . . He had the switchblade at my breasts and kept asking if he could "slice one for a souvenir" . . .
>
> . . . He stood straddling me and urinated up and down my body, to "warm me up." I threw up and he turned my face over into it and penetrated me anally again, pressing my face into the vomit. I didn't have to hold my breath that time. I just passed out from sheer terror.
>
> (Easteal & McOrmond Plummer, 2006, p. 73)

## Obsession

The obsessive rapist shares similar aspects with the sadist, but his arousal is fueled less by causing suffering and torment, and more by specific perverse acts he forces his partner to engage in (Finkelhor & Yllo, 1985; Martin et al., 2007). Perpetrators are preoccupied with certain types of sex acts that may be bizarre or unusual. They may read and/or watch pornography and write or talk extensively about their obsession:

> . . . he had this pinup on the wall above our bed, and he turned around and ripped my clothes off and all the rest of it, and raped me . . . There were heaps of pinups but this one particular one he looked at and he would turn around and get the biggest carrots that he could get, like at the supermarket or cucumbers or the salamis and he would be ramming them up me . . .
>
> (Easteal & McOrmond Plummer, 2006, p. 75)

It is unimportant to an obsessive rapist if his partner is willing to participate in fantasy play. And he may be completely unperturbed by the pain his actions have caused. One woman, anally raped so frequently that she developed health problems, says:

I had explained to him that the act itself did nothing for me sexually, nor emotionally, and that physically it had awful side-effects. And it never changed his actions towards me. His preference and pleasure came before concern for me.

(Easteal & McOrmond Plummer, 2006, p. 76)

## Myths that perpetrators may act out

IPSV perpetrators may be acting out false beliefs about masculinity, male sexuality, and rape. They may also be using them to justify their violence. We review a few of these myths in order to help the reader to be able to confront or penetrate their denial.

### Men who rape their partner are out of control

Carol Adams writes, "Men who abuse and rape their partners are men who seek to control others. In being abusive they are not out of control; rather, they establish control" (Adams, 1993, p. 68). Yet, there persists the common belief that rape is the act of a man out of control of his emotions or sexual urges. Understanding that perpetrators do choose to rape, and that they have control over their deeds, contradicts that myth (McOrmond-Plummer, 2014).

My awareness of his intent to use rape in a deliberate way became clearer as I allowed myself to reflect on how he spoke to me in the course of sexual violence: "I am going to hurt you," "There's only one way to teach you not to be a whore;" "Just try and stop me, you bitch." . . . a specific outcome in mind by somebody who knew he was using sex in a controlling and controlled way.

(Easteal & McOrmond Plummer, 2006, p. 77)

The partner who uses verbal coercion to maneuver his partner into unwanted sex is also behaving with awareness. He hears, "No," or some other signal of unwillingness, but proceeds to manipulate the emotions of his partner until he gets what he wants. He knows that she has fears or other vulnerabilities and he capitalizes on them. Consider the following words of a man who admitted to the emotional coercion of his wife: "I would act like I was mad at her and she would give in. It works every time" (Hite, 1981, p. 749). This is not the behavior of a man out of control; it is a man taking control.

### Rape is part of "manhood"

From Greek mythology of raping gods, to wars in which the prize for the victorious is the right to rape the women on the conquered side, and on to present-day videogames that award points to players who capture and rape an electronic "victim," rape is depicted as the act of conquerors and heroes.

Some men think rape equates with virility and power. It may be seen as a means of putting women "in their place" – that is, beneath men. For example, a woman whose partner raped her while a friend of his was present, says,

> [He] had needed to prove himself as a real man, one worthy of membership in his friend's group. My violation was his proof of who wore the trousers. I don't think I will ever forgive the culture of masculinity for working against me and other women in the terrible way it has.
>
> (Easteal & McOrmond Plummer, 2006, p. 78)

### Sex is the normal entitlement of men in a relationship

Some women report that following IPSV, their partner may behave as if he has not done anything wrong – perhaps due to a belief that it is his right to have sex with his partner: "I think he saw it as a part of our relationship that was normal. Being entitled to sex with me as his girlfriend played a role definitely" (Easteal & McOrmond Plummer, 2006, p. 80). There are persisting sexist social values that support such beliefs: "Macho" men were also more likely to believe in the concept of "wifely duty" and that men were justified in using force (Martin, Taft & Ressick, 2007, p. 339).

Sex with a partner is seen as the *entitlement* of men (Pence & Paymar, 1993). This myth is widely supported; one man was advised by a psychiatrist to rape a wife who withheld sex (Russell, 1990). According to this view, women who withhold sex from their partners should interpret rape as a natural outcome of nonconsent. He'd say, "Your body's my body and I want to look at my body so I'm quite entitled" (Easteal & McOrmond Plummer, 2006, p. 35).

See Chapter 5 for more on entitlement.

### Rape is a type of making love

Diana Russell (1975, pp. 110–111) writes, "Some rapists think they're lovers." These men are likely to subscribe to myths that women want a forceful lover, or that women like being raped. "No" isn't heard as withdrawing consent, but is seen as part of a game the perpetrator has every intention of winning – in fact the word "No" may be heard as "No, I want you to force me." There might be initial attempts at verbally persuading a woman to have sex, but the underlying intention is to do it anyway. To these men, consent is nice but not a necessity.

Some survivors of IPSV describe their partners as treating the rapes as legitimate sexual encounters. Rape may be normalized by the perpetrator as "making love"; afterwards, he may be attentive and affectionate.

He stripped me naked in the lounge and raped me, having picked me up by my breasts from behind and dragged/carried me to the settee. Afterward, while I was getting dressed, and trying to light a cigarette with shaking hands, he made me a cup of coffee, then sat down next to me to drink his, as though we had just made love.

(Easteal & McOrmond Plummer, 2006, p. 81)

## Conclusion

We hope to have shed light in this chapter upon common motivations for sexual assault and rape, and myths that men who rape their partners may subscribe to. Challenge to notions of who rapes and why is essential, particularly since partner rape is often wrongly conflated with sex, rather than the act of violence that it is (McOrmond-Plummer, 2014). It is most important that the partner rapist is not given a free pass because he may have had a consensual relationship with his victim. An understanding of the mindset that underpins IPSV will also be an asset to those working with abusers.

## References

Adams, C. (1953). "I just raped my wife! What are you going to do about it, Pastor?" The Church and sexual violence. In E. Buchwald, P. Fletcher, & M. Roth (Eds.), *Transforming a rape culture*. Minneapolis, MN: Milkweed Editions.

DeKeseredy, W. (2014). Separation/divorce sexual assault. In L. McOrmond-Plummer, P. Easteal, & J.Y. Levy-Peck (Eds.), *Intimate partner sexual violence: A multidisciplinary guide to providing services and support for survivors of rape and abuse* (pp. 65–75). London, UK: Jessica Kingsley Publishers.

Easteal, P., & McOrmond-Plummer, L. (2006). *Real rape, real pain: Help for women sexually assaulted by male partners*. Melbourne, Australia: Hybrid Press.

Englander, E. (2003). *Understanding violence*. Mahweh, NJ: Lawrence Erlbaum.

Finkelhor, D., & Yllo, K. (1985). *License to rape: Sexual abuse of wives*. New York, NY: The Free Press.

Frances, A., & Wollert, R.J. (2012). Sexual sadism: Avoiding its misuse in sexually violent predator evaluations. *Journal of the American Academy of Psychiatry and the Law*, 40(3), 409–416.

Groth, A., & Birnbaum, H. (1979). *Men who rape: The psychology of the offender*. New York, NY: Plenum Press.

Hite, S. (1981). *The Hite Report on male sexuality: How men feel about love, sex, and relationships*. New York, NY: Knopf/Random House.

Holmes, R.M., & Holmes, S.T. (2002). Psychological profiling and rape. In R.M. Holmes & S.T. Holmes (Eds.), *Profiling violent crimes: An investigative tool* (3rd ed.) (pp. 139–157). Thousand Oaks, CA: Sage.

Hucker, S.J. (1997). Sexual sadism: Psychopathology and theory. In R. Laws & W. O'Donohue (Eds.), *Sexual deviance: Theory, assessment and treatment* (pp. 194–209). New York, NY: Guilford Press.

Kelly, J., & Johnson, M. (2008). Differentiation among types of intimate partner violence: Research update and implications for interventions. *Family Court Review*, 46(3), 476–499.

Leone, J., Johnson, M., & Cohan, C. (2007). Victim help seeking: Differences between intimate terrorism and situational couple violence. *Family Relations, 56,* 427–439.

McOrmond-Plummer, L. (2014). Considering the differences: Intimate partner sexual violence. In L. McOrmond-Plummer, P. Easteal, & J.Y. Levy-Peck (Eds.), *Intimate partner sexual violence: A multidisciplinary guide to providing services and support for survivors of rape and abuse* (pp. 41–51). London, UK: Jessica Kingsley Publishers.

Martin, E., Taft, C., & Resick, P. (2007). A review of marital rape. *Aggression and Violent Behavior, 12,* 329–347.

Pence, E., & Paymar, M. (1993). *Education groups for men who batter: The Duluth Model.* New York, NY: Springer.

Russell, D. (1975). *The politics of rape: The victim's perspective.* New York, NY: Stein & Day.

Russell, D. (1990). *Rape in marriage.* New York, NY: Macmillan Publishing Company.

Shapcott, D. (1988). *The face of the rapist.* Auckland, New Zealand: Penguin Books.

# Chapter 5

# Intimate partner sexual violence perpetrators and entitlement

*Debra Parkinson*

## Introduction

> Q. What kind of man rapes his wife?
> A. Any man. Normal men.
>
> (Michael Flood, 2009, 1:16)

In the absence of a perpetrator profile, male entitlement is at the root of IPSV. We necessarily begin with the gender hierarchy, male power and violence, and the cultural attachment to marriage and the nuclear family.

The social construction of gender identifies that men are taught to expect more of everything (Austin, 2008; Connell, 2005; Pease, 2010). Men have more power and choice, higher status, and greater wealth: "Where we are is deep inside an oppressive gender legacy, faced with the knowledge that what gender is about is tied to a great deal of suffering and injustice" (Johnson, 2005, p. 4).

Domination of women, violence, and abuse serve to uphold male privilege and traditional manhood (Pease, 2012). Even in the twenty-first century, outdated notions of men's conjugal rights and sexual double standards persist – shored up by new technologies which bring fresh opportunities to oppress and shame women (Henry & Powell, 2015). Theories drawn from feminist and masculinity scholarship identify the ways that male privilege is established and sustained. One framework points to three pillars: (1) male control of institutions; (2) cultural ideals of masculinity and devaluing of women; and (3) that men's experiences come to represent human experiences (Johnson, 2005). The greatest perpetuator of male privilege is its apparent normality, its invisibility. In essence, "the fish do not know the water is wet" (Allen, 2002, p. 192). Where discrimination is recognized, there are countless and subtle ways that defenders of patriarchy ward off claims for equality from women, including denial and examples of individual men suffering (Johnson, 2005). Judith Allen (2002) writes: "Inherently unstable, masculinity is always in process, under negotiation, needing to be 'shored up,' reinforced, buttressed against its many enemies" (p. 199).

Research by Willer, Rogalin, Conlon, and Wojnowicz (2013) confirms the theory of "masculine overcompensation," whereby men demonstrate a kind of hyper-masculinity to counter their insecurity. Their research identifies hormonal involvement in men's responses, confirming earlier observations of the use of violence by men when their privileged position is threatened (Pease, 2012). For men who are marginalized and fail to meet the stringent standards of the ideal man, violence may be their only advantage (Austin, 2008) and domination over the women close to them may result (Coston & Kimmel, 2012; Pease, 2010). bell hooks observes that men "believe that their identity can be gained through the oppression of another, specifically women" (cited in Austin, 2008, p. 10), and Anna Goldsworthy (2013, p. 13) writes that, "Violence is the last resort of the disenfranchised man: if trumped by a woman, he can still fall back on brute strength." This chapter extends the concept of male privilege and entitlement to consider the way it plays out in intimate partner sexual violence (IPSV). It does this through the words of women, health professionals, and police officers who participated in research on partner rape in Victoria, Australia, in 2008, and concludes with strategies to challenge the underpinning male sense of entitlement.

## Existing research

There are few consistent research findings on IPSV perpetrator characteristics beyond that perpetrators are overwhelmingly men (Breiding et al., 2014; Martin, Taft, & Resick, 2007). They are a diverse group, with no common profile of a "husband-rapist" (Bergen & Barnhill, 2011; Purdie, Abbey, & Jacques-Tiura, 2010). Perpetrators are often violent in other ways (Bennice & Resick, 2003; Coker, Smith, McKeown, & King, 2000; Martin, Taft, & Resick, 2007; Purdie, Abbey, & Jacques-Tiura, 2010); however, IPSV may also be the only form of violence perpetrated by male partners (Bergen & Barnhill, 2011). In their 2007 review of marital rape literature, Martin and colleagues concluded that IPSV perpetrators commonly hold more power and status than their partners and tend to be hostile toward women, believing in their right to be dominant and their right to marital and impersonal sex (Martin, Taft, & Resick, 2007). Belief in entitlement is reiterated as a key characteristic by other researchers (Purdie, Abbey, & Jacques-Tiura, 2010; Raquel & Bukovec, 2006). Beyond these points, there are few consistent characteristics. The effect of variables such as family of origin, sexual characteristics, unemployment, and alcohol and drug use is contested, with studies reporting contrasting findings (Martin et al., 2007).

## Methodology

Women's Health Goulburn North East (WHGNE) conducted qualitative research in 2008, with Upper Murray Centre Against Sexual Assault (UMCASA) assisting with interviews, and acting as a critical friend. In-depth, semi-structured interviews were held with 21 women, and a combination of interviews and focus groups were conducted with 23 health professionals and 30 police officers in Victoria, Australia. Ethics approval was granted and interviews recorded and transcribed. Analysis was based on Glaser and Strauss's Grounded Theory (1967).

Criteria for inclusion were that women had to be aged over 18 and to have named their experience as rape by a former husband or intimate partner. In the sample of women, the age range was 27–70. Four were Aboriginal and two were migrants. For five women, the rapes were recent with two cases before the courts. For the other 16 women, the rapes took place more than 5 years earlier, but were still raw in their impact. Participants were recruited through flyers at women's services and advertisements in local newspapers.

## Findings

### Perpetrators: Who are they?

The men described by the 21 women were diverse. They included men employed at high levels and men who were unemployed. While some men fit the stereotype of the violent and recognizable abuser, most did not. Two were outstanding citizens, recognized with awards by their communities. Many were "good looking," "smooth talkers," "nice guys," financially well-off. Sexual assault survivors have reported the same charming attributes in perpetrators who could suddenly become ominous, threatening, and dangerous – a kind of "Dr. Jekyll and Mr. Hyde" change (Clark & Quadara, 2010, p. 38). Likewise, women in this research spoke of a hidden side to their partner, which in some cases only emerged after many years of marriage. According to Anne: "I don't know what's happened, I don't understand him at all. When I was doing my annulment I realised how little I knew him. It was scary. How can you be married to someone and not know them?" Elizabeth said: "It keeps coming to me – the look on his face, it was like it wasn't him. I now see a different side of him to who I was married to."

As with Clark & Quadara's (2010) respondents, some described the men's sexual activity as "queer," "perverse," "bizarre," or "fantasy-land." They described how their husbands had affairs, used prostitutes, raped them after watching pornography, "moulded" them into sex objects for their use, and insisted on sexual activity that the women found unacceptable (see also Chapter 2 for similar behaviors on the part of lethal abusers and Chapter 13 for more on perpetrators' use of pornography). Anne disclosed: "I think maybe he was feeling inadequate because of the pornography and then tried to project that on to me . . . Maybe because I wasn't performing as in the porn? Because he had bags and bags of porn."

One woman said her husband was generally unable to have sex, with the exception of sex for procreation and for the one incident of rape years after the end of the marriage. Victoria explained:

He was unable to have sex. Ordinarily he couldn't have sex, I remember the dates of the three children being conceived. There was never gratuitous sex. There was just never sex. The moment I was pregnant, I went almost 18 months before he touched me again. He was never that sort of man.

Another would only rape – there was never consensual sex. Some had sexually abused children and one had raped a young woman with an intellectual disability.

Insecurity was identified as a problem with some of the men. The women reflected on the apparent inferiority felt by their partners because of differences in education level or popularity and social standing, and thought they used rape as proof of their masculinity and superiority. Marcia explained: "Funnily enough, I think too that he had an inferiority complex because I actually had a very good education, and he left school at 14." Janet described her experience: "Rape is their proof of their masculinity and their power over you. Their dominance. It's a primeval thing. You are my property."

Some women suggested that men who rape their wives and partners have sometimes been raised to think they have a right to do as they want with a woman; that women are there to be used, to meet their needs and to do what they're told. Two women described their mothers-in-law as blaming them and actively trying to prevent them from seeking help.

Others reflected that perhaps love and nurturing were absent from their partners' childhoods and they consequently felt neglected and rejected as children. One woman wondered if it was the molesting of her partner as a young boy by his uncle that led to his violent and sexually abusive treatment of her. According to Anne: "I think there was a lot of basic loving and nurturing missing from his life. I think he's sought other things."

Elizabeth explained:

He's got a lot of hang-ups about his mother and about me because I'm a strong woman. He has no respect for women, he goes off with floosies. He apparently has no self-confidence but he's pretty good looking, and financially OK.

In an attempt to make sense of this behavior, some women considered their ex-husbands to be mentally ill, suggesting diagnoses such as sociopathy, schizophrenia, and depression.

One man resented his own babies for taking what was his. He demanded anal sex because he stated childbirth had stretched his wife's vagina too much, and his resentment went further because one child had a health problem which took his wife's time and energy.

Men were described as angry and bad tempered; as verbally and emotionally abusive; as financially abusive; as controlling in every area of daily life. These men seemed to believe they had a right to control what their wife or partner did. Fraser explained: "It started to snowball, to 'I want and I'll have'." Laura recalled how "One night he brought out the marriage certificate and said, 'I've got a piece of paper that says you do as I say.'"

Louise described her experience of being controlled:

> In six years I wasn't allowed to have any money, I wasn't allowed to drive a car, everywhere I went he went with me and I wasn't allowed out of the house, and if I didn't answer the phone he would be on the doorstep within an hour saying "Where were you?" So there was huge control, huge control.

Three-quarters of the women interviewed described that violence played a role in addition to the rapes they suffered. The spectrum of violent behavior included threats to kill the woman and her children, gross physical violence, stabbing, and an axe attack. "[He] used to threaten to kill me throughout the marriage; and more recently, in February, just before moving into my house, he threatened to kill me twice within a week" (Anne). "He knows I'm frightened of him. I'm afraid if I took a stand he will hurt me. The only day that will make me happy is when he is dead" (Sarah).

Janet had a terrifying experience:

> My first husband used to like oral and anal sex. I didn't like either so he smashed me in the face so I had to have all my teeth out and he could force oral sex. He could force any bloody thing he wanted to. It's just violence to prove that they are big and strong and you are nothing.

While drugs and alcohol were factors identified by twelve women as contributing to their husbands' behavior, a strong theme emerging from the research is that the kind of man who rapes his wife or partner takes advantage of those less "powerful" than himself. The women pointed to their own times of vulnerability which were coldly exploited. They spoke of when they were sick with epilepsy, severe disability, mental illness, cancer, or broken bones; or when they were unconscious, pregnant or with a new baby; when they were very young and unsupported by family; when they were purposely isolated by their husband from family and friends either geographically or socially. One Aboriginal woman was enticed from her family at 17 and, six months later, the abuse began. Vulnerability occurred, too, through lack of financial resources and through strong religious faith. The men we heard about in this research took advantage of all these vulnerabilities. According to Julia:

> At the time that I met [him] I was really not in a mentally right state. I should have been seeing a psychiatrist or psychologist or should have been in a hospital really. He got me at a weak moment and he wouldn't leave and I ended up getting pregnant.

And Sarah described how "I was only young at the time and he was a lot older. He was 31 and my experience of sex before that wasn't much. He thought he might train me. I was 17."

### Men's sense of entitlement to sex

All of the 21 women stated that 23 of the 24 men would not have named their actions as rape. This is the most bewildering finding of the research. Yet, according to the legal definition, all 21 women were raped. We know that 17 women said no. One woman was unconscious and one was drugged. One chose between a rape and a beating. One could not remember saying no because she is affected by posttraumatic stress disorder.

A total of 17 of the 21 women reported other kinds of violence in their relationship concurrent with the rapes. One woman, Fraser, had her back broken while being anally raped. Another, Laura, thought she would die when her husband held a pillow over her face "combined with a couple of hits around the head" while raping her. Anne had cancer and described how her husband would keep pushing and pushing and she could feel the cancer. She would cry with pain. Monique and Juana were held captive by their partners. Monique was stabbed seven times when he found her at the railway station trying to escape. Victoria was victim to an elaborately planned attack when, after eight years' separation she was raped by her ex-husband. He had taken Viagra in order to complete the rape and had enticed her to the house with the excuse that he needed to discuss the children.

How could these men apparently not see their action as rape? One woman thought it was because her partner considered his behavior as acceptable "in his own mind"; for one man, perhaps because he saw sex as a mixture of pleasure and pain; for several men, because it was her fault; for most men because he had done nothing wrong – they were married, she was "his," it was normal, it was his sexual appetite. "He absolutely would not recognise this action as rape. No. Never, never. Even if he's found guilty and put away, he'll go to his grave believing this is my fault" (Victoria). "He says I made him do it. He's not going to take responsibility for what he's done" (Jacqui). "They're the man, they're the boss in the relationship so you do what I say. So I don't think he would have seen it as rape. He would have seen me as his property and he could do as he wanted" (Juana).

Even when women confronted their husband or partner, the men's reactions were universally to deny the rape. "I said to him, 'That's what you done' and he just sort of giggles it off. You say it again to him and it's seriously like he doesn't think in his own head that he's done anything wrong" (Monique). "He didn't think there was anything wrong with doing what he did. 'All men do that.' He said, 'You're my wife. We had sex.' He doesn't recognise it as rape" (Elizabeth).

"No, he doesn't [recognise his actions as rape]. I've had this discussion with him, and no, he totally denies everything and doesn't believe he did a thing to this day" (Louise).

A uniformed officer agreed: "No, men would not call their actions rape, they would classify it as their right. If they had to be 100% honest they'd say, 'I did take advantage of her but stuff it, she's my missus anyway, it's Saturday night.'"

### Society's complicity in the male sense of entitlement to marital sex

By silencing women through undermining their experience or disbelieving them, or by regarding the institution of marriage as more worthy of our respect than an individual's human rights, we conspire with the men who rape their partners. As family members, friends, ministers of religion, doctors and police, we excuse them. Rurality exacerbates the complicity and patriarchy that work together to tolerate – if not nurture – a culture of violence against women. We heard that police, church ministers and doctors knew what was happening and did nothing. And worse, that women who spoke up suffered recriminations from their community. A health professional told us: "One woman in a small country town was raped very badly by her husband. She told the local minister and the local police about it and they counselled her to keep her mouth shut" (HP 9).

As Raquel Kennedy Bergen (1995) writes: "women have historically lacked a social definition that allowed them to see the abuse as anything more than a personal problem." As discussed in Chapter 14, the legal response also reflects society's ambivalent view of the seriousness of IPSV.

## How to challenge men's sense of entitlement to women's bodies

### Address gender inequality and remove gender stereotypes

According to VicHealth, "the most significant determinants of violence against women are the unequal distribution of power and resources between men and women [and] an adherence to rigidly defined gender roles" (VicHealth, 2011, p. 1). The two are entwined as strict gender roles, which largely determine the kind of work that can be undertaken with women restricted by the primary caregiver role (Pocock, Charlesworth, & Chapman, 2013; AHRC, 2013).

Male/female as a binary category is the basic defining feature of Australia and other similar countries, and levels of discrimination against women vary as starkly outlined in the UN's ranking (World Economic Forum, 2014). The dichotomy, however, is itself flawed, and a blunt instrument with which to assign gendered roles. Transgender, genderqueer, and other individuals reject traditional categorization. Biologically, too, there are genetic, hormonal, and anatomical variants from the male and female "norm," such as people who identify as intersex.

A shift away from this inaccurate categorization of individuals into one of two tick boxes indicating "male" or "female" is an important step in challenging men's entitlement to women's bodies. The status quo that positions men as more entitled and more privileged is immediately undermined by a spectrum of ways of being. No longer automatically assigned to male and female roles, children can become the individuals they aspire to with a range of possibilities and role models. Progress in this direction has been made in the Scandinavian countries as they take all five of the top positions in gender equality (World Economic Forum, 2014). In Australia, the Australian Human Rights Commission (AHRC, 2013) and the Workplace Gender Equality Agency have a raft of strategies to promote cultural change for equal participation and reward of men and women in employment.

### Challenge the sexual double standard

Its existence remains undeniable, as innumerable insults for women's bodies and sexual expression sit alongside a yawning absence of such slurs for men – the few that are used refer to feminine or homosexual tendencies (girly, gay) or their mothers (son of a bitch, bastard) rather than to the male himself. Insults pertaining to a small penis and impotence reiterate the demand for men to be "real" men. No moral double-bind exists for men in the way it is framed for women. The notion of "Madonna" or "whore" (Conrad, 2006; Summers, 1994) condemns women either way. Shame continues to belong to women (Weiss, 2010), as indicated by continued victim-blaming, facilitated as it is by twenty-first century technologies (Henry & Powell, 2015).

Two key strategies are early education on respectful relationships directed to boys and girls at school (see also Chapter 21), and ongoing media and Internet campaigns to challenge male physical and sexual violence and privilege. Police officers interviewed offered their insight on both strategies, and one officer said that education for males is needed to teach "that females are not just a piece of equipment to be used whenever you want it."

### Name the problem

Braaf (2011) concluded that victims of partner rape are vulnerable both to repeated assaults and to homicide. It is deeply concerning that many health professionals continue their reluctance to name the problem. Both time- and resource-poor, they need to be persuaded, first that partner rape is prevalent, seriously damaging, and a crime; and second that an effective response can be feasible and fast with referral information (Parkinson & Reid, 2014).

### *Hold men to account for partner rape*

The myths that surround partner rape can be exposed through open and public discussion that is informed by feminist theory and scholarship on men and masculinities. Its criminality can be upheld by prosecuting and sentencing perpetrators of partner rape and through alternatives such as restorative justice (Daly, 2011).

## Conclusion

The perpetrators of partner rape are indeed normal men, any man. The women who informed this research described 24 perpetrators of IPSV and their descriptions spanned the gamut of ages, education, occupations, class, wealth, status and personality. Some men chose to perpetrate this violence on their wife or intimate partner from the start and regularly. Two waited, and the sexual assaults followed decades of happy marriage. Women described partners variously using sexual violence to assert some definition of "masculinity"; to punish them or seek retribution; to indulge in their fantasies of violent sex; to satisfy sadistic urges; or to put their woman in her place. For some, it was simply that he wanted sex and it was her job as a wife to provide it. He had "a piece of paper to prove it." The predatory nature of their attacks was clear in many of the women's accounts, from the "carer" who began his assaults after marrying his seriously disabled wife, to the man whose first attack was when his wife was in bed with a broken ankle, to the man whose assaults on his pregnant wife caused her late miscarriage. In these cases, men exploited their opportunity and greater power.

Male privilege is a defining feature of our society and men's sense of entitlement to sex with female partners is deeply entrenched. Despite the illegality of rape and sexual violence in intimate relationships, legal consequences for perpetrators are rare. Health professionals and community members commonly minimize women's concerns or entirely neglect the issue. The effect is to leave women alone with this hidden and heartbreaking problem – one that has been linked to a greater risk of femicide (Braaf, 2011). Critically, the effect is also to leave men's entitlement intact. As Bob Pease (2008) writes about violence, although we may not be perpetrators, we are *perpetuators* when we do nothing and say nothing. By pretending partner rape does not exist, we are complicit in its remaining unnoticed and uncensored.

## References

AHRC (2013). *Investing in care: Recognising and valuing those who care* (Vol. 1: Research Report). Sydney, Australia: Australian Human Rights Commission.

Allen, J.A. (2002). Men interminably in crisis? Historians on masculinity, sexual boundaries, and manhood. *Radical History Review, 82*(Winter), 191–207.

Austin, D.W. (2008). Hyper-masculinity and disaster: Gender role construction in the wake of Hurricane Katrina. Paper presented at the American Sociological Association Annual

Meeting, Boston, MA. Retrieved from: www.allacademic.com/meta/p241530_index. html.

Bennice, J.A., & Resick, P.A. (2003). Marital rape: History, research, and practice. *Trauma, Violence and Abuse, 4,* 228–246.

Bergen, R.K. (1995). Surviving wife rape: How women define and cope with the violence. *Violence Against Women, 1*(2), 117–138.

Bergen, R.K., & Barnhill, E. (2011). *Marital rape: New research and directions.* Harrisburg, PA: National Resource Center on Domestic Violence (NRCDV).

Braaf, R. (2011). Preventing domestic violence death – is sexual assault a risk factor? (Research and Practice Brief). Sydney, Australia: Australian Domestic and Family Violence Clearinghouse. Retrieved from: www.adfvc.unsw.edu.au/PDF%20files/Research_&_ Practice_Brief_1.pdf.

Breiding, M.J., Smith, S.G., Basile, K.C., Walters, M.L., Jieru, C., & Merrick, M.T. (2014). Prevalence and characteristics of sexual violence, stalking, and intimate partner violence victimization – National Intimate Partner and Sexual Violence Survey, United States, 2011. *MMWR Surveillance Summaries, 63*(8), 1–18.

Clark, H., & Quadara, A. (2010). *Insights into sexual assault perpetration* (Research Report No. 18). Melbourne, Australia: Australian Institute of Family Studies.

Coker, A.L., Smith, P.H., McKeown, R.E., & King, M.J. (2000). Frequency and correlates of intimate partner violence by type: Physical, sexual, and psychological battering. *American Journal of Public Health, 90*(4), 553–559.

Connell, R.W. (2005). *Masculinities* (2nd ed.). Los Angeles, CA: University of California Press.

Conrad, B. (2006). Neo-institutionalism, social movements, and the cultural reproduction of a mentalité: Promise keepers reconstruct the Madonna/whore complex. *Sociological Quarterly, 47*(2), 305–331.

Coston, B.M., & Kimmel, M. (2012). Seeing privilege where it isn't: Marginalized masculinities and the intersectionality of privilege. *Journal of Social Issues, 68*(1), 97–111.

Daly, K. (2011). Conventional and innovative justice responses to sexual violence. *ACSSA Issues* (12), 1–35.

Flood, M. (2009). Partner rape: Know about it, respond effectively, prevent it (video file). Wangaratta, Australia: Women's Health Goulbourn North East. Retrieved from: www.whealth.com.au/work_partner_rape.html.

Glaser, B., & Strauss, A. (1967). *The discovery of grounded theory: Strategies for qualitative research.* Chicago: Aldine.

Goldsworthy, A. (2013). Unfinished business: Sex, freedom and misogyny. *Quarterly Essay, 50*(June), 1–76.

Henry, N., & Powell, A. (2015). Beyond the 'sext': Technology-facilitated sexual violence and harassment against adult women. *Australian & New Zealand Journal of Criminology, 48*(1), 104–118.

Johnson, A. (2005). Where are we? In A. Johnson (Ed.), *The Gender Knot* (pp. 3–26). Philadelphia, PA: Temple University Press.

Martin, E.K., Taft, C.T., & Resick, P.A. (2007). A review of marital rape. *Aggression and Violent Behaviour, 12,* 329–347.

Parkinson, D., & Reid, S. (2014). "Invisible" intimate partner sexual violence: Prevention and intervention challenges. In L. McOrmond-Plummer, P. Easteal, & J.Y. Levy-Peck (Eds.), *Intimate partner sexual violence: A multidisciplinary guide to improving services and support for survivors of rape and abuse* (pp. 136–146). London, UK: Jessica Kingsley Publishers.

Pease, B. (2008) *Engaging Men in Men's Violence Prevention: Exploring the Tensions, Dilemmas and Possibilities* (Issues Paper 17). Sydney, Australia: Australian Domestic and Family Violence Clearinghouse. Retrieved from: www.adfvc.unsw.edu.au/PDF%20files/Issues%20Paper_17.pdf.

Pease, B. (2010). *Undoing privilege: Unearned advantage in a divided world*. London, UK: Zed Books.

Pease, B. (2012). The politics of gendered emotions: Disrupting men's emotional investment in privilege. *Australian Journal of Social Issues, 47*(1), 125–142.

Pocock, B., Charlesworth, S., & Chapman, J. (2013). Work–family and work–life pressures in Australia: Advancing gender equality in "good times"? *International Journal of Sociology and Social Policy, 33*(9/10), 594–612.

Purdie, M.P., Abbey, A., & Jacques-Tiura, A.J. (2010). Perpetrators of intimate partner sexual violence: Are there unique characteristics associated with making partners have sex without a condom? *Violence Against Women, 16*, 1086–1097.

Raquel, K.B., & Bukovec, P. (2006). Men and intimate partner rape: Characteristics of men who sexually abuse their partner. *Journal of Interpersonal Violence, 21*(10), 1375–1384.

Summers, A. (1994). *Damned whores and God's police* (2nd ed.). Melbourne, Australia: Penguin.

VicHealth (2011). *Preventing violence against women in Australia: Research summary addressing the social and economic determinants of mental and physical health*. Carlton, Australia: Victorian Health Promotion Foundation.

Weiss, K. (2010). Too ashamed to report: Deconstructing the shame of sexual victimization. *Feminist Criminology, 5*(3), 286–310.

Willer, R., Rogalin, C.L., Conlon, B., & Wojnowicz, M.T. (2013). Overdoing gender: A test of the masculine overcompensation thesis. *American Journal of Sociology, 118*(4), 980–1022.

World Economic Forum (2014). Global gender gap report 2014. Retrieved from: http://reports.weforum.org/global-gender-gap-report-2014/rankings/.

# Perpetrators of intimate partner sexual violence

## Characteristics, motivations, and implications for assessment and intervention

*Joseph A. Camilleri and Melissa M. Miele*

## Introduction

As with any criminal behavior, the causes of intimate partner sexual coercion are likely complex and multifaceted. This chapter focuses exclusively on the characteristics and motivations of perpetrators of intimate partner sexual violence (IPSV), which, relative to other areas of sexual and domestic violence, have been given little scholarly attention. Camilleri and Quinsey (2009a) reported that only 2% of the psychological literature on sexual coercion focused exclusively on partner sexual coercion. Work on intimate partner sexual violence has not kept up with the increase in research on sexual assault in general, possibly due to perceptions that IPSV is not as problematic as other forms of sexual violence (see Attitudes and Perceptions, this chapter).

## Defining intimate partner sexual violence

IPSV includes all forms of sexual aggression and coercion in intimate, committed relationships. The phrase intimate partner sexual violence treats violence in a broader context to include verbal actions and risk for psychological harm (Washington Coalition of Sexual Assault Programs, 2016), and is consistent with how "intimate partner violence includes violence more broadly" (Black et al., 2011). In this chapter, we use a general definition of IPSV, which is "any sexual act against a committed intimate partner that may result in psychological or physical harm." IPSV therefore includes couples who are in a marital, engaged, or enduring dating relationship. Other terms that capture sexual offending in the context of conjugal, committed, or courting relationships include forced in-pair copulation (Goetz & Shackelford, 2006), partner rape (forced sex against an unwilling partner), and partner sexual coercion (coerced sex with an unwilling partner).

## Characteristics of perpetrators

Few studies have considered the characteristics of IPSV perpetrators. Early work on understanding IPSV perpetrators asked victims to describe conditions associated with IPSV, which included some information about perpetrators. For example, Finkelhor and Yllo's (1985) survey of women's experience with IPSV collected some information on their partners' demographics, and found, for example, that the highest prevalence rates were from the lowest family income bracket (24%). Using a smaller follow-up sample, they gathered additional information on types of sexual acts, sources of conflict, and other demographic/historic information and reported that the major source of conflict was sex (49% reported). Money (29%), drinking (27%), children (27%), and jealousy (27%), all were close for the second most common conflict issue. Other variables were reported, but it was unclear whether they were attributes of the perpetrator, victim, or both.

Other early studies reported similar descriptive information on demographics, assumed motivation, perceived dominance characteristics, views on wife abuse, and jealousy (Bergen, 1996; Campbell & Alford, 1989; Mahoney & Williams, 1998; Russell, 1990). Though important in understanding the scope of this problem, these results should be treated as an initial glimpse into the characteristics and motivations of perpetrators and not as an exhaustive description of perpetrators, due to the potential response bias from victims (e.g., Finkelhor & Yllo, 1985; Ullman & Siegel, 1993) and proneness of qualitative methods to experimenter bias (e.g., Bergen, 1996; Russell, 1990). Also, there were no clear theoretical frameworks guiding hypothesis development, which is not too surprising considering these early works were exploratory. One way to better understand etiology is to see if IPSV perpetrators share characteristics with other offenders, or if their characteristics are unique in some ways.

## Categorizing intimate partner sexual violence

Many offenders are categorized based on crime type and relationship to the victim. Perpetrators of IPSV are somewhat unique in that they can be categorized as either sexual offenders or partner assaulters (Camilleri & Quinsey, 2009a), which is an important consideration since there is very little overlap in these literatures. Intimate partner violence and sexual offenders have their own assessments, causal theoretical explanations, and characteristics, which begs the question: *Are IPSV offenders more similar to sexual offenders or to partner abusers, or are they unique in terms of their psychological profile?* Camilleri and Quinsey (2009a) compared a sample of rapists, partner rapists, and partner assaulters, on paths to general antisocial behavior, which included age (younger men typically account for a larger proportion of crimes), developmental incidents (individuals with developmental setbacks have an increased probability of crime), and psychopathy (a personality trait associated with many types of criminal behavior).

They also compared these groups on criminal history and risk of violent recidivism. Overall, there is no pattern to suggest partner rapists resemble either group – they are more similar to rapists on psychopathy, more similar to partner assaulters in terms of criminal history, similar to both on age and IQ, and dissimilar to both on risk to commit a violent reoffense. In other words, using factors associated with general criminality, there is no indication that partner rapists can easily be included into another general crime type. Further support for this conclusion is that where significant differences are observed, the size of the differences is rather large, suggesting that partner rapists are not just different, but very different on certain variables relative to comparable offender groups.

Note that it is possible that these samples may vary on how representative they are because they came from a forensic psychiatric institution. For instance, there is the possibility that partner rapists are rarely ever charged or convicted – rape in general is largely unreported (Langton, Berzofsky, Krebs, & Smiley-McDonald, 2012; Kruttschnitt, Kalsbeek, & House, 2014), suggesting IPSV is under-reported to a greater degree – which means that only the most severe cases end up in the criminal justice system.

## Individual differences

What motivates or increases the probability of IPSV may depend on variation among men in traits that are either causally related to IPSV or are associated with antisocial behavior (i.e., rule breaking). Here we review traits that may be directly or indirectly associated with IPSV, including psychopathy and attitudes toward rape.

### Psychopathy

Psychopaths are individuals whose personality is oriented toward using others for personal gain. Conceptually, psychopaths have been thought of as social predators (Book, Quinsey, & Langford, 2007; Hare, 2001), whereby their personality traits assist and maintain exploitative behavior, and whose cognitive abilities are enhanced when it comes to identifying and remembering people who are exploitable (Book, Costello, & Camilleri, 2013; Camilleri, Kuhlmeier, & Chu, 2010). Psychopaths can also be understood as sexual predators – not only is psychopathy a significant predictor of sexual recidivism (Hanson & Morton-Bourgon, 2005), current theoretical and empirical evidence supports the possibility that coercive, precocious, and elevated sexuality are fundamental characteristics of being a psychopath (Harris, Rice, Hilton, Lalumière, & Quinsey, 2007). If such is the case, we might expect these traits to impact psychopaths' sexual interaction with partners.

Theoretically, psychopathy has more recently been considered an alternative life-history strategy with an orientation toward risky, egocentric behaviors that are costly to others. In ancestral environments, such a "cheater" strategy would have conferred survival and reproductive benefits, as long as there were not many people with such traits in a population (Mealey, 1995). Whereas most men are prone to engage in risky behavior after they reach puberty and desist as they mature and age, psychopaths appear to have an alternative trajectory. This group shows early signs of antisocial behavior, has very high rates of violent recidivism, commits more severe types of crimes, and continues to engage in such behaviors at a high rate well into adulthood, though burnout seems to occur after 40 years of age (Hare, McPherson, & Forth, 1988; Lalumière, Mishra, & Harris, 2008). Although much is known about psychopathic traits, correlates, and consequences, very little is known about the nature of intimate relationships for these men.

Much of the research that considered consequences of psychopaths in relationships has focused on intimate partner nonsexual violence (IPV), with a number of studies finding strong associations between psychopathy and IPSV. Hilton et al. (2001) studied men convicted of assaulting their partner. Although wife assaulters as a group had lower psychopathy scores than other offenders, psychopathy still significantly predicted violent recidivism. In another sample, Hilton et al. (2001) identified psychopathy as not just the strongest predictor of wife assault recidivism, but also a predictor of the number of recidivistic incidents, severity of victim injury, and number of severe incidents. Because of the strength of the Psychopathy Checklist-Revised's association with recidivism, it was included as part of an in-depth actuarial risk assessment, the *Domestic Violence Risk Appraisal Guide* (Hilton, Harris, Rice, Houghton, & Eke, 2008). Other studies have considered various ways in which psychopathy is related to intimate partner violence (Fowler & Westen, 2011; Harris, Hilton, & Rice, 2011; Stanford, Houston, & Baldridge, 2008), and researchers are now studying its clinical role, such as psychopathy's impact on batterer treatment failure (Rock, Sellbom, Ben-Porath, & Salekin, 2013).

Considering psychopathy is a robust predictor of many different types of crimes, including partner assault and sexual assault, Camilleri and Quinsey (2009a) tested to see if it is also associated with IPSV. Using a self-report assessment of psychopathy from a sample of community and student participants, Camilleri and Quinsey (2009a) found that scores correlated with self-reported propensity for partner sexual coercion. Recognizing the limitations of self-report, Camilleri and Quinsey also conducted an archival study of convicted partner rapists, and found that 33% qualified as having a diagnosis of psychopathy (which was not significantly different from the proportion of psychopathic rapists: 54%) – that is, about a third of convicted partner rapists met the diagnostic criteria for psychopathy.

### Attitudes and perceptions

Attitudes, which are positive and/or negative evaluations of an object (Eagly & Chaiken, 1998), are an interesting area of psychology related to IPSV because of the possible link between attitudes and behavior, and because modifying attitudes may prevent, to some degree, sexually violent behavior. Even though men generally have more positive attitudes toward marital rape, a significant proportion of women also share such views (e.g., Monson, Langhinrichsen-Rohling, & Binderup, 2000). How attitudes manifest in behavior may therefore be moderated by sex. For example, among women, attitudes supportive of marital rape may minimize victims' interest in pursuing criminal charges, whereas among men, it may increase the risk of engaging in such behavior.

The relevant question for this chapter is whether variation in attitudes is associated with variation in IPSV behavior. Little attention has been given here. In fact, we could not locate any studies that looked at marital rape attitudes held by men who had committed such acts. A method that most closely linked partner-rape perceptions to behavior used a measure of self-perceived interest in using either coaxing or coercive tactics to obtain sex from a reluctant sexual partner, and found that it correlated with self-reported frequency and severity of partner sexual coercion (Camilleri, Quinsey, & Tapscott, 2009). A strong sex difference was demonstrated from a significant correlation between perceived interest in partner sexual coercion and the Sexual Coercion in Relationships Scale among men, not among women; the correlation with the sexual coercion subscale of the Conflict Tactics Scale, however, was not significant for either men or women. These results provide some encouraging, although not overwhelming, evidence linking attitudes with behavior. Attitude research with men convicted of such behavior would be a logical next step.

## Environmental conditions

Unlike individual differences, the impact of environmental conditions on IPSV is understood as a facultative trigger whereby the risk of engaging in such behavior is increased under particular conditions.

### Sexual jealousy

Sexual jealousy, whether a result of suspected or actual partner infidelity, has been a robust predictor or component of conflict in intimate relationships (Buss, 2000). Similar to other variables associated with IPSV, sexual jealousy was initially empirically linked with nonsexual IPV and domestic homicide (Hilton et al., 2001, 2004; Wilkinson & Hamerschlag, 2005; Wilson & Daly, 1996).

Camilleri and Quinsey (2009b) found that a majority of partner rapists (72%) experienced some degree of suspected or actual partner infidelity or loss of partner to another man. Although this proportion was not significantly different from that of partner assaulters, partner rapists experienced significantly more jealousy-provoking events than did partner assaulters. Other studies found similar patterns: direct cues to partner infidelity were more strongly associated with sexual victimization from a partner than nonsexual physical victimization

(Miele & Camilleri, 2011), and partner rapists reported the highest levels of partner infidelity – partner assaulters reported lower levels and nonoffender controls reported the lowest levels (Shields & Hanneke, 1983).

One specific type of jealousy-provoking event, relationship dissolution, is a commonly observed condition prior to committing IPSV (Bergen, 1996, as cited in Mahoney & Williams, 1998; Finkelhor & Yllo, 1985, as cited in Mahoney & Williams, 1998). Some 9% of Camilleri and Quinsey's (2009b) partner rapist sample had a partner who had left or planned to leave the relationship.

Not all of these studies have clearly delineated between actual and suspected infidelity, so it is possible that men also vary on the degree to which they get jealous. We would therefore expect men who score higher on measures of jealousy, or are pathologically jealous (also called morbid jealousy and delusional disorder-jealous type), are at a higher risk of partner sexual violence. Much of the literature has found an association between morbid jealousy and IPSV (Easton & Shackelford, 2009; Silva, Ferrari, Leong, & Penny, 1998). Though no studies on delusional jealousy have looked at its association with IPSV, we expect to find particularly strong associations here as well.

## *Alcohol*

Alcohol consumption is not just implicated in general sexual offending (e.g., Abbey et al., 2001) and intimate partner violence (Barnett & Fagan, 1993; O'Leary & Schumacher, 2003), but there is some evidence to suggest it is associated with IPSV as well (reviewed in Martin et al., 2007). Alcohol use is implicated more in sexual than in nonsexual violent behavior (Abracen, Looman, & Andersen, 2000), but whether such patterns also emerge in intimate relationship violence is unknown. Alcohol abuse (or any substance abuse) does not predict sexual recidivism (Hanson & Bussiere, 1998), but we could not identify any studies looking at alcohol's impact on IPSV recidivism.

Perpetrator alcohol use, not victim alcohol use, predicted sexual offending severity across all types, and victim/perpetrator drinking is more implicated in cases where the victims do not know the perpetrator very well (Ullman & Brecklin, 2000). Other findings are mixed in terms of the effects of people's use of alcohol (reviewed in Mahoney & Williams, 1998); some studies found high alcohol use by victims of IPSV prior to victimization (Zablotska et al., 2009). Still, the association between alcohol use and IPSV is understudied; therefore, strong conclusions cannot be made.

## Typology of partner rapists

A common research question is whether perpetrators of a particular act can be organized into meaningful "types," commonly referred to as a *typology*. Accurate criminal typologies can be useful because they elucidate paths to behavior, which should inevitably inform its prevention. Several typologies of IPSV exist to categorize behaviors (Finkelhor & Yllo, 1985), sexual interests (Russell, 1990), or dimensions that are difficult to discern (Monson & Langhinrichsen-Rohling, 1998; Proulx & Beauregard, 2014). Given the paucity of research on IPSV perpetrators, a surprising amount of attention has been given to categorizing IPSV, and so several concerns with currently available typologies should be noted:

1. Some typologies are informed either by sexual offender typologies or by batterer typologies, but partner rapists may be a unique offender category. It is not clear whether they are a subset of either general group.
2. No overarching theory predicts or explains any of these IPSV typologies, or was used to inform their measurement.
3. Separate types were informed by separate theories (e.g., Monson & Langhinrichsen-Rohling, 1998).
4. Data supporting typologies were mostly from victims.
5. No clear implications are stated as to how typologies can be used for clinical intervention or public safety through prevention.
6. Each vary on what they are categorizing (behaviors, victim type, sexual motivation).
7. Not clear whether types are supposed to be static (i.e., once in category, always in a category) or dynamic (i.e., can shift in and out of any category).
8. None explain the large sex difference found in IPSV perpetration and victimization.
9. Some samples were small and included women.
10. Use of cluster analyses (statistical methods for grouping subjects) to develop types are inappropriate because they are inductive, and do not accurately test hypotheses of types (Schmidt, Kotov, & Joiner, 2004).
11. Cluster analytic techniques are generally problematic for several reasons: There are no appropriate methods to validate group assignment through cluster analysis; such methods are quite poor at determining group membership; there are no criteria to determine which cluster analytic methods to use (Schmidt et al., 2004); rules to determine the number of clusters are highly problematic (Ruscio, Haslam, & Ruscio, 2006).

## Evolutionary typologies

A more meaningful approach to typology research is to first identify an appropriate dimension from which "types" are determined. Using an evolutionary approach to classify offenders based on etiology may be useful because it considers both *ultimate causes* of behavior (e.g., variation in trait associated with variation in fitness benefits) and their *proximate causes* (i.e., IPSV developmental trajectory and environmental triggers; Nesse, 2013). Camilleri (2012) used such an evolutionary approach to identify a typology of sexual offenders based on ultimate causes of sexually aggressive behavior, whereby sexual offending could exist as an adaptation (trait designed to increase fitness), a byproduct of an adaptation (trait that does not confer reproductive success, but is a byproduct of trait(s) that do), or as a disordered adaptation (trait due to malfunctioning adaptation). Each type is based on these different etiological paths. Camilleri and Quinsey (2012) summarized the literature on two possibly adaptive paths to partner rape: cuckoldry risk and psychopathy. IPSV may be considered a byproduct when it is followed by uxoricide (murder of a wife by her husband), and IPSV as a disorder could occur among men with intellectual disabilities or delusional jealousy (Camilleri, 2012). Interestingly, other traits we reviewed, such as attitudes, perceptions, and alcohol use, can be thought of as proximal mechanisms of these other paths.

Nonevolutionary typologies focus on proximate causes, but any single trait associated with sexual offending can have different causes or developmental trajectories. Thus, the evolutionary psychological approach is more comprehensive because it considers types based on both ultimate and proximate causes. This approach may also provide theoretical unity across previous work on IPSV typologies because many characteristics associated with sexual crimes (e.g., anger, sadism, cognitive distortions, attitudes, alcohol) can be thought of as proximal causes (i.e., how, psychologically, would someone be more prone to sexually assaulting a partner), whereas types are dependent on ultimate causes (i.e., answers why a person would sexually assault a partner).

This latter step is needed because proximal causes alone do not explain why negative affect, for example, is associated with sexual offending (Proulx, Beauregard, Lussier, & Leclerc, 2014). Many people experience anger, contempt, and disgust, but do not sexually offend, so additional circumstances and conditions, informed by ultimate causes, are needed to fully understand causation. Also, women experience these conditions but they rarely sexually offend. Taking an evolutionary approach may provide a useful framework in understanding complex interactions of variables associated with sexual and relationship conflict (Camilleri, 2012; Camilleri & Quinsey, 2012; Camilleri & Stiver, 2014).

## Implications for assessment and treatment

As we reviewed, some similarities exist between IPSV offenders and other types of offenders, including domestic violence and sex offender groups, so one approach to treating IPSV offenders is to modify currently available programs for IPSV/batterers. A more effective approach, however, is to design sexual offender treatment based on criminogenic needs that are unique to offender types, including IPSV offenders (Camilleri, 2012).

Assessment and treatment should be guided by Andrews et al.'s (1990) principles of effective correctional programming. Their meta-analysis found that programs targeting risk (i.e., those who are at high risk to recidivate), criminogenic need (i.e., changeable traits associated with recidivism), and responsivity (i.e., conditions that improve receptivity to programming) showed the greatest impact on recidivism. Thus, assessment of offender risk, need, and responsivity of IPSV perpetrators are required to guide intervention. Moving forward, treatment for IPSV offenders should focus on offenders who are at high risk (with special attention and research on psychopathic offenders), should target specific need areas (sexual jealousy, attitudes, and alcohol consumption) and should focus on combating Factor 1 psychopathy traits to improve responsivity (see Olver, Lewis, & Wong, 2013).

## Summary and conclusions

This chapter was designed to provide a comprehensive framework for understanding perpetrators of intimate partner sexual violence, particularly their characteristics and motivations, and how this research would inform assessment and treatment. Navigating this literature is difficult because different terms and definitions are used, which complicates research on IPSV prevalence, causes, and consequences. Though IPSV perpetrators share some characteristics with sexual offenders and batterers, they do not clearly fit in either category, and should be examined as an independent group. There have been meaningful developments in identifying different types of IPSV perpetrators. An evolutionary framework may provide theoretical unity in all domains of IPSV research and practice because it integrates both ultimate and proximate causes. Three major characteristics associated with IPSV perpetration include psychopathy, sexual jealousy, and alcohol abuse, though additional traits may emerge with theoretical and empirical developments. Understanding the characteristics, conditions, typology, and motivations of IPSV perpetrators has important implications for assessment and intervention, particularly practice that is guided by risk, need, and responsivity principles of effective correctional programing. We hope that our framework will provide researchers and clinicians a helpful blueprint when dealing with this problematic behavior.

## References

Abbey, A., Zawacki, T., Buck, P., Clinton, A.M., & McAuslan, P. (2001). Alcohol and sexual assault. *Alcohol Research & Health, 25*(1), 43–51.

Abracen, J., Looman, J., & Anderson, D. (2000). Alcohol and drug abuse in sexual and nonsexual violent offenders. *Sex Abuse, 4,* 263–274.

Andrews, D.A., Zinger, I., Hoge, R.D., Bonta, J., Gendreau, P., & Cullen, F.T. (1990). Does correctional treatment work? A clinically relevant and psychologically informed meta-analysis. *Criminology, 28*(3), 369–404.

Barnett, O.W., & Fagan, R.W. (1993). Alcohol use in male spouse abusers and their female partners. *Journal of Family Violence, 8*(1), 1–25.

Bergen, R.K. (1996). *Wife rape: Understanding the response of survivors and service providers* (Vol. 2). Thousand Oaks, CA: Sage Publications.

Black, M.C., Basile, K.C., Breiding, M.J., Smith, S.G., Walters, M.L., Merrick, M.T., Chen, J. & Stevens, M.R. (2011). *The National Intimate Partner and Sexual Violence Survey (NISVS): 2010 summary report.* Atlanta, GA: National Center for Injury Prevention and Control, Centers for Disease Control and Prevention.

Book, A.S., Quinsey, V.L., & Langford, D. (2007). Psychopathy and the perception of affect and vulnerability. *Criminal Justice and Behavior, 34*(4), 531–544.

Book, A., Costello, K., & Camilleri, J.A. (2013). Psychopathy and victim selection: The use of gait as a cue to vulnerability. *Journal of Interpersonal Violence, 28,* 2368–2383.

Buss, D.M. (2000). *The dangerous passion: Why jealousy is as necessary as love and sex.* New York, NY: Simon & Schuster.

Camilleri, J.A. (2012). Evolutionary psychological perspectives on sexual offending from etiology to intervention. In T.K. Shackelford & V.A. Weekes-Shackelford (Eds.), *Oxford handbook of evolutionary perspectives on violence, homicide, and war* (pp. 173–196). New York, NY: Oxford University Press.

Camilleri, J.A., & Quinsey, V.L. (2009a). Individual differences in the propensity for partner sexual coercion. *Sexual Abuse: A Journal of Research and Treatment, 21*(1), 111–129.

Camilleri, J.A., & Quinsey, V.L. (2009b). Testing the cuckoldry risk hypothesis of partner sexual coercion in community and forensic samples. *Evolutionary Psychology, 7*(2), 164–178.

Camilleri, J.A., & Quinsey, V.L. (2012). Sexual conflict and partner rape. In A.T. Goetz & T.K. Shackelford (Eds.), *Oxford handbook of sexual conflict in humans* (pp. 257–268). New York, NY: Oxford University Press.

Camilleri, J.A., & Stiver, K.A. (2014). Adaptation and sexual offending. In T.K. Shackelford & V.A. Weekes-Shackelford (Eds.), *Evolutionary perspectives on human sexual psychology and behavior* (pp. 43–67). New York, NY: Springer.

Camilleri, J.A., Quinsey, V.L., & Tapscott, J.L. (2009). Assessing the propensity for sexual coaxing and coercion in relationships: Factor structure, reliability, and validity of the tactics to obtain sex scale. *Archives of Sexual Behavior, 38*(6), 959–973.

Camilleri, J.A., Kuhlmeier, V.A., & Chu, J.Y.Y. (2010). Remembering helpers and hinderers depends on behavioral intentions of the agent and psychopathic characteristics of the observer. *Evolutionary Psychology, 8*(2), 303–316.

Campbell, J.C., & Alford, P. (1989). The dark consequences of marital rape. *The American Journal of Nursing, 89*(7), 946–949.

Eagly, A.H., & Chaiken, S. (1998). Attitude structure and function. In D.T. Gilbert, S.T. Fiske, & G. Lindzey (Eds.), *The handbook of social psychology* (pp. 269–322). Boston, MA: McGraw-Hill.

Easton, J.A., & Shackelford, T.K. (2009). Morbid jealousy and sex differences in partner-directed violence. *Human Nature, 20,* 342–350.

Finkelhor, D., & Yllo, K. (1985). *License to rape: Sexual abuse of wives.* New York, NY: Simon & Schuster.

Fowler, K.A., & Westen, D. (2011). Subtyping male perpetrators of intimate partner violence. *Journal of Interpersonal Violence, 26*(4), 607–639.

Goetz, A.T., & Shackelford, T.K. (2006). Sexual coercion and forced in-pair copulation as sperm competition tactics in humans. *Human Nature, 17*(3), 265–282.

Hanson, R.K., & Bussiere, M.T. (1998). Predicting relapse: A meta-analysis of sexual offender recidivism studies. *Journal of Consulting and Clinical Psychology, 66,* 348–362.

Hanson, R.K., & Morton-Bourgon, K.E. (2005). The characteristics of persistent sexual offenders: a meta-analysis of recidivism studies. *Journal of Consulting and Clinical Psychology, 73*(6), 1154–1163.

Hare, R.D. (2001). Psychopaths and their nature: Some implications for understanding human predatory violence. In A. Raine & J. Sanmartín (Eds.), *Violence and Psychopathy* (pp. 5–34). New York, NY: Springer.

Hare, R.D., McPherson, L.M., & Forth, A.E. (1988). Male psychopaths and their criminal careers. *Journal of Consulting and Clinical Psychology, 56*(5), 710–714.

Harris, G.T., Rice, M.E., Hilton, N.Z., Lalumière, M.L., & Quinsey, V.L. (2007). Coercive and precocious sexuality as a fundamental aspect of psychopathy. *Journal of Personality, 21*(1), 1–27.

Harris, G.T., Hilton, N.Z., & Rice, M.E. (2011). Explaining the frequency of intimate partner violence by male perpetrators: Do attitude, relationship, and neighborhood variables add to antisociality? *Criminal Justice and Behavior, 38*(4), 309–331.

Hilton, N.Z., Harris, G.T., & Rice, M.E. (2001). Predicting violence by serious wife assaulters. *Journal of Interpersonal Violence, 16*(5), 408–423.

Hilton, N.Z., Harris, G.T., Rice, M.E., Lang, C., Cormier, C.A., & Lines, K.J. (2004). A brief actuarial assessment for the prediction of wife assault recidivism: The Ontario domestic assault risk assessment. *Psychological Assessment, 16*(3), 267–275.

Hilton, N.Z., Harris, G.T., Rice, M.E., Houghton, R.E., & Eke, A.W. (2008). An indepth actuarial assessment for wife assault recidivism: The Domestic Violence Risk Appraisal Guide. *Law and Human Behavior, 32*, 150–163.

Kruttschnitt, C., Kalsbeek, W.D., & House, C.C. (2014). *Estimating the incidence of rape and sexual assault.* Washington, DC: National Academies Press.

Lalumière, M.L., Mishra, S., & Harris, G.T. (2008). In cold blood: The evolution of psychopathy. In J. Duntley & T.K. Shackelford (Eds.), *Evolutionary forensic psychology: Darwinian foundations of crime and law* (pp. 139–159). New York, NY: Oxford University Press.

Langton, L., Berzofsky, M., Krebs, C., & Smiley-McDonald, H. (2012). *Victimizations not reported to the police, 2006–2010.* Special Report – National Crime Victimization Survey. Washington, DC: U.S. Department of Justice.

Mahoney, P., & Williams, L.M. (1998). Sexual assault in marriage: Prevalence, consequences, and treatment of wife rape. In *Partner violence: A comprehensive review of 20 years of research* (pp. 113–163). Thousand Oaks, CA: Sage.

Martin, E.K., Taft, C.T., & Resick, P.A. (2007). A review of marital rape. *Aggression and Violent Behavior, 12*(3), 329–347.

Mealey, L. (1995). The sociobiology of sociopathy: An integrated evolutionary model. *The Behavioral and Brain Sciences, 18*(03), 523–541.

Miele, M.M., & Camilleri, J.A. (2011). Understanding paths to sexual and physical violence in relationships. Presented at the Poster Presented at the 2nd North American Correctional and Criminal Justice Psychology Conference, Toronto, Canada.

Monson, C.M., & Langhinrichsen-Rohling, J. (1998). Sexual and nonsexual marital aggression: Legal considerations, epidemiology, and an integrated typology of perpetrators. *Aggression and Violent Behavior, 3*(4), 369–389.

Monson, C.M., Langhinrichsen-Rohling, J., & Binderup, T. (2000). Does "no" really mean "no" after you say "yes"? Attributions about date and marital rape. *Journal of Interpersonal Violence, 15*(11), 1156–1174.

Nesse, R.M. (2013). Tinbergen's four questions, organized: A response to Bateson and Laland. *Trends in Ecology & Evolution, 28*(12), 681–682.

O'Leary, K.D., & Schumacher, J.A. (2003). The association between alcohol use and intimate partner violence: Linear effect, threshold effect, or both? *Addictive Behaviors, 28*(9), 1575–1585.

Olver, M.E., Lewis, K., & Wong, S.C.P. (2013). Risk reduction treatment of high-risk psychopathic offenders: The relationship of psychopathy and treatment change to violent recidivism. *Personality Disorders*, *4*(2), 160–167.

Proulx, J., & Beauregard, E. (2014). Pathways in the offending process of marital rapists. In J. Proulx, E. Beauregard, P. Lussier, & B. Leclerc (Eds.), *Pathways to Sexual Aggression* (pp. 110–136). New York, NY: Routledge.

Proulx, J., Beauregard, E., Lussier, P., & Leclerc, B. (2014). *Pathways to sexual aggression.* New York, NY: Routledge.

Rock, R.C., Sellbom, M., Ben-Porath, Y.S., & Salekin, R.T. (2013). Concurrent and predictive validity of psychopathy in a batterers' intervention sample. *Law and Human Behavior*, *37*(3), 145–154.

Ruscio, J., Haslam, N., & Ruscio, A.M. (2006). *Introduction to the taxometric method: A practical guide.* Mahwah, NJ: Lawrence Erlbaum Associates.

Russell, D.E.H. (1990). *Rape in marriage.* Bloomington, IN: Indiana University Press.

Schmidt, N.B., Kotov, R., & Joiner, T.E., Jr. (2004). *Taxometrics: Toward a new diagnostic scheme for psychopathology.* Washington, DC: American Psychological Association.

Shields, N.M., & Hanneke, C.R. (1983). Battered wives' reactions to marital rape. In D. Finkelhor, R.J. Gelles, G.T. Hotaling, & M.A. Straus (Eds.), *The dark side of families* (pp. 131–148). Beverly Hills, CA: Sage.

Silva, A.J., Ferrari, M.M., Leong, G.B., & Penny, G. (1998). The dangerousness of persons with delusional jealousy. *The Journal of the American Academy of Psychiatry and the Law*, *26*(4), 607–623.

Stanford, M.S., Houston, R.J., & Baldridge, R.M. (2008). Comparison of impulsive and premeditated perpetrators of intimate partner violence. *Behavioral Sciences & the Law*, *26*, 709–722.

Ullman, S.E., & Brecklin, L.R. (2000). Alcohol and adult sexual assault in a national sample of women. *Journal of Substance Abuse*, *11*(4), 405–420.

Ullman, S.E., & Siegel, J.M. (1993). Victim–offender relationship and sexual assault. *Violence and Victims*, *8*(2), 121–134.

Washington Coalition of Sexual Assault Programs (2016). Intimate partner sexual violence. Retrieved from: www.wcsap.org/intimate-partner-sexual-violence.

Wilkinson, D.L., & Hamerschlag, S.J. (2005). Situational determinants in intimate partner violence. *Aggression and Violent Behavior*, *10*(3), 333–361.

Wilson, M.I., & Daly, M. (1996). Male sexual proprietariness and violence against wives. *Current Directions in Psychological Science*, *5*(1), 2–7.

Zablotska, I.B., Gray, R.H., Koenig, M.A., Serwadda, D., Nalugoda, F., Kigozi, G., Sewankambo, N., Lutalo, T., Mangen, F.W., & Wawer, M. (2009). Alcohol use, intimate partner violence, sexual coercion and HIV among women aged 15–24 in Rakai, Uganda. *AIDS and Behavior*, *13*(2), 225–233.

# Chapter 7

# What type of men sexually assault their partners, and why do women love them?

## Beyond stereotyping

*Louise McOrmond-Plummer*

## Introduction

Enduring myths about rape and domestic violence include notions about the "type" of man who commits these crimes. These myths often take the form of believing that "nice" men cannot be rapists, and vice versa – that rapists can never be nice men. The belief that neither proposition is possible leads to assumptions that are inaccurate and harmful. It is essential that practitioners intersecting with survivors, or with perpetrators themselves, challenge stereotypes they may hold about who commits rape. Many people also do not understand how or why women love men who sexually abuse them. It is just as important that such women are not negatively stereotyped. This chapter looks at both of these often misunderstood areas.

## Quandaries

Writing this chapter was a challenge. Given the danger to women that perpetrators of IPSV represent, does it really matter that they can be "nice guys" when they're not being abusive? Isn't focusing on their abusive behavior a priority? And isn't there trouble enough with the family and friends of a perpetrator dissuading his victim from seeking safety by telling her how wonderful he is, and even parading into the courts to do the same, as if, for example, being a pillar of the Church preempts committing rape? Of course, it is also a fact that many abusers are "nice" in order to manipulate their partners, or family and friends (Bancroft, 2003). On the other hand, the popular view of rapists is that they are complete reprobates, forever defined by their crimes. However, for reasons that will become apparent, this view creates problems when dealing with victims/survivors or perpetrators of IPSV.

## Can perpetrators of IPSV be nice men?

The short answer to this question is that perpetrators of rape and other abuse can indeed be nice men – in appearance or in reality. In many cases, they have qualities with which women fall in love, and which may hold women in relationships with them:

> He was the one who was originally interested in me, and I was flattered, so agreed to date him. We found out how much we liked each other, and how much fun we had together, and we became a couple. We adored each other, and were very compatible in a lot of ways. We both liked the same activities, and laughed a lot. Much of our time was spent going to movies, dancing, visiting friends, going to Halloween parties and dressing in weird costumes, going through the water parks or on the roller coasters in the pouring rain, going to the zoo and making faces at the animals, or just hanging out.
>
> ("Natalie," Easteal & McOrmond-Plummer, 2006, p. 85)

## Why does taking into account positive aspects of IPSV perpetrators matter?

In more than a decade of managing my website, Aphrodite Wounded, I have received correspondence from many survivors of IPSV, and also occasionally from men who have raped their partners. Some time ago, a man identifying as "Keith" contacted me with an admission that he had raped his wife, and expressed seeming sorrow at his actions. I am always dubious when I receive such correspondence, because there is no way that I, being just a woman behind a computer screen, can ascertain whether it is genuine, or if the man's partner is safe. Abusers can be skilled manipulators, and I have no desire to collude with them in manipulating their partners. In general, I do not reply to them. Nevertheless, it was at least possible that Keith may have been genuine, and I was interested in conversing with some friends and colleagues on social media about his letter, in order to get the benefit of their perspectives.

One woman seemed infuriated by any positive conjecture about Keith's motives. She held the view that rapists are bad people beyond redemption, and that my refusal to agree with her that they are unmitigated bastards signified that I had more compassion for perpetrators than for survivors, and indeed, constituted a *betrayal* of survivors. Finally, she suggested that I should bake baskets of muffins for rapists! I did feel somewhat upset about these accusations at the time. However, balance was regained upon reflection that in my experience, many survivors of partner rape require not only empathy for the fact that they were sexually assaulted, but also understanding and acceptance that the very partners who raped them can be good people when they are not being abusive. They are often anxious that people understand that their partners have positive aspects. For example, a woman may report that the partner who assaulted her is a good father, easy to talk to, a hard worker or an excellent lover. And, occasionally, women report that their partners have taken genuine steps to cease sexual and other abuse (Easteal & McOrmond-Plummer, 2006).

Thus, to have agreed with the woman's position would have been the true betrayal of the survivor group I would like my work to serve. Meeting survivors wherever they are emotionally, and being willing to hear any positive feelings they may have for their abusers is basic respect, and is absolutely mandatory when dealing with women who have had respect taken away from them by sexual or other violence.

For many survivors of IPSV, an important part of healing, empowerment, and ending the violence is giving their violations the name of "rape," and the perpetrator the name of "rapist" (Russell, 1990; Bergen, 1996; Easteal & McOrmond-Plummer, 2006). In a society that all too frequently waters down IPSV as not "real" rape, it is essential that professionals do not collude with silence and minimization around partner rape. Even so, survivors will often state that the sexual assaults do not constitute the whole of their relationships; neither does "rapist" define their partner in entirety.

With respect to the view of men who have raped as intractably evil, it is surely possible – and from a professional point of view, *necessary* – to recognize a whole person without absolving him of responsibility for abuse. For example, in a correspondence about the present work, Rus Ervin Funk, co-author of Chapters 13 and 17, stated his preference for referring to perpetrators as *men who have perpetrated violence* (McOrmond-Plummer, 2014, personal communication). I appreciate the way this differentiates between people and their actions. Those who work with "men who have perpetrated violence" will undoubtedly recognize this as a useful position.

However, discussions about positive aspects of perpetrators are not intended to indicate that because an abuser can be good sometimes, sexually abusing his partner does not matter. While a woman must be heard when she speaks about the positive aspects of her partner, she must also hear that it is never okay for anybody to sexually assault her. When an abuser attempts to minimize the abuse by maximizing any positive things that he does – as they frequently do (Bancroft, 2003) – he must hear that even if these things are true, sexually assaulting his partner is unacceptable. These discussions also make no case for minimizing the danger of IPSV to women, especially when we reflect that even where there are positive times, men who combine rape of their partners with battery are more likely to murder them (see Adams, Chapter 2).

## Problems with taking "niceness" of perpetrators at face value

Lundy Bancroft (2003) writes at length about the ability of abusers to turn on gold-plated charm for their partner, her friends, family, and anybody who may intervene. Narcissistic or psychopathic abusers with no empathy or conscience are capable of exhibiting charm that may fool even shrewd judges of character, including seasoned counselors. So, if somebody who has raped or otherwise abused his partner is capable of being loving to her at different times, the question is whether it is genuine, or if he is using it as simply another tool of control. For example, is he trying to get his partner to reconcile? It is often at this time that women get the most passionate avowals of love, gifts, unusual spates of help with children, and promises of change (Herman, 1992). In this case, the "niceness" is simply another form of abusive control.

Some perpetrators do actually love their partners (Matsakis, 1996). Apologies for abuse may, in the moment, be quite genuine. Unfortunately, many of these men are unwilling to back up their words with action and make real change to their behavior. Because they derive benefit from having power over women, they do not ultimately want to relinquish it (Bancroft, 2003). The primary issue here for professionals is not whether the abuser actually loves his partner, but her safety. It is interesting to consider how an abuser may define "love" – for example, it may mean possession (see Chapter 10).

In his practice, Bancroft (2003) has observed that "Mr. Sensitives" (that is, men who appear to be very sensitive, gentle, and who talk the right talk about respecting women), may in fact be abusive, but because people don't believe these men are "the type," they are able to conceal it more successfully. And many men who enjoy more traditionally masculine pursuits such as football and hunting are not necessarily more likely to be abusive than the "Mr. Sensitives."

## Can nice men be perpetrators of IPSV?

The question posed earlier in this chapter was whether perpetrators of sexual assault can be nice men. In this section, I reverse that question and use as a starting point the perceived "niceness" of the perpetrator. Readers will note the nuances in both questions.

Janice Yap (a woman from my hometown) had been married for 25 years when her husband David, a well-known local businessman and member of several charity organizations, began drugging and sexually assaulting her (Cooke, 2008). The ensuing welter of letters to the media expressing anger for pillorying this "good man" was perhaps not particularly surprising when we consider the eagerness of many people to believe that "good men" cannot be perpetrators of sexual assault. Only two letters – from one other woman and myself – appeared in support of Ms. Yap, who showed truly impressive courage and persistence in defending the truth despite the praise and sympathy heaped upon her husband (and the loss of access to grandchildren). While David Yap was convicted and fined for indecently assaulting his wife, the conviction was not recorded because the magistrate took pity on the embarrassment he had suffered.

When actor Bill Cosby, renowned for his harmlessly avuncular brand of humor, was accused of drugging and raping several women, his wife, Dr. Camille Cosby, released a public statement (CBS Evening News, 2014) that the man the media was talking about was a man she did not know; her husband of decades was a loving, kind, and wonderful husband. Lynn Beisner's (2014) open letter in reply to Dr. Cosby eloquently made the point that her husband may, in truth, be all of those positive things *and* still be a rapist.

With respect to partner rape, it is common for women to describe their partners as having a "Jekyll and Hyde personality." While there is a higher likelihood of a batterer using sexual assault as another form of abuse, not all partner rapists are habitually violent, and in fact their relationships may even appear to be otherwise egalitarian. For example, survivor Natalie says: "It did not occur to me until just one year ago, about 14 years after the rape, that it HAD been rape. I always said he had attacked me, but found it very difficult to see him as a rapist. There was absolutely no indication in the seven years of our relationship that he could be violent, and I know he adored me" (Easteal & McOrmond-Plummer, 2006, p. 111).

Many people hold notions about rapists as tattooed strangers in alleyways who have psychiatric issues; a rapist is not the nice man next door who gives you vegetables from his garden. Yet, partner rapists are generally quite ordinary men (Russell, 1990). Survivor Kuriah says, "The majority of the time it was a normal existence. We spent time with his friends, took our son to the park, went on vacation, bought things for the house, made slow sensual love. But over time things changed more and more" (Easteal & McOrmond-Plummer, 2006, p. 88). After Kuriah and her husband split, her husband – this man who could be an otherwise loving partner – raped and beat her in an attack that almost killed her (Easteal & McOrmond-Plummer, 2006).

## Why do "nice" men rape their partners?

We have seen that men are capable of raping their partners no matter how nice or normal they may seem. It is beyond the scope of this chapter to describe comprehensively why men rape, but one significant aspect is *mindset*. The mindset of men who rape their partners may comprise several factors, such as sexual entitlement (see Chapter 5), and subscription to rape myths, such as "It's not rape if it's your partner." "Nice" men may carry these common and socially ingrained beliefs, and thus be a risk to their partners (see Chapter 4 for a more in-depth discussion on the mindset of IPSV perpetrators, and myths they may subscribe to).

## What about perpetrators who are rarely or never nice to their partners?

There are abusers who appear to have very few qualities that could be described as positive. Their sole purpose in taking up with a female partner appears to be that of unrelenting abuse, contempt, and violence. For example, in an Australian case (Silkstone, 2004), Graeme Slattery lent a woman some money, after which they became lovers, and she moved to Slattery's property to carry out some work to pay off the financial debt. Slattery kept the woman in a garage and subjected her to a host of sexual and other tortures which make truly horrifying reading, including (in a move redolent of the dehumanization of slavery and concentration camps) taking his victim's name away and forcing her to have his chosen name of "Toerag" tattooed on her arm. Even so, Slattery's charm was still sufficient, at least initially, to engage this woman to become his lover, and later for him to convince the police, whom a neighbor had called after *witnessing Slattery kicking and punching the woman*, that his victim had problems with medication.

Further, my website contains accounts from women and teenage girls whose partners evidently did not even pretend to express any love or kindness toward them. They have, among other things, been set up for gang rape by their partners, defecated upon, pimped, and blackmailed with threats of their children being sexually abused for noncompliance with their partners' demands. What a woman sees as "positive" in these cases may be simply being allowed to eat, not being beaten, or not having to work the streets for a night because she is ill. Another example of almost unabated abuse was Victor Burnham, who, among other things, allegedly forced his wife to have sex with the family dog (Russell, 1990). Also, there are situations that may not involve constant physical violence and degradation, but are characterized by lengthy patterns of emotional cruelty (for example, see Jodie's story in Easteal and McOrmond-Plummer, 2006).

## Why do women love men who rape them?

In exploring the crime of marital rape and the question of why women remain with perpetrators, sex-crime researchers Holmes and Holmes (2002) list reasons such as fear of reprisal or removal of children, after which they add, "In talking with some marital rape victims, we were surprised that one additional reason, and a popular one, was that the spouse still loved the partner rapist!" (pp. 231–232). The exclamation mark perhaps conveys a kind of quizzical shock on the part of the authors. It is common for people not to comprehend why women profess love for men who abuse them, and at worst, this leads to women being stigmatized as "sick," or blamed for the abuse. However, to anybody who has worked with domestic violence – including IPSV – a woman's ongoing love for the perpetrator is neither surprising nor particularly shocking. I have already discussed some of the reasons above. It is crucial for professionals to be able to hear about a woman's reasons for loving her abuser.

Victims of violence experience the effects of abuse and trauma, which may lead to them professing love and loyalty for an abuser after even the most severe betrayals. The following factors provide some explanation:

### Stockholm syndrome

This takes its name from a bank robbery and five-day hostage situation which took place in Sweden in 1973. Upon release, the hostages professed empathy and even love for their captors, some offering to raise money for their captors' legal defense. Stockholm Syndrome may be applicable to numerous situations, including domestic violence, in which, for an array of psychological reasons, cruel treatment binds victim to perpetrator (Herman, 1992).

## Traumatic bonding

Traumatic bonding occurs as a result of cycles of violence, in which beatings, rape, and other mistreatment are mixed with kindness, love, or even extending the most basic rights such as a meal or allowing the victim to use the toilet. Abused women learn that the same person who harms them is also a source of comfort. Many survivors know what it is to sink gratefully into the arms of an abuser who is offering comfort after a beating and/or rape – it can feel quite literally as if the perpetrator is all the woman has. He is being kind when she feels incredibly vulnerable and it does not matter that *he caused* the vulnerability.

Traumatic bonding may also be fueled by a woman's hope for the future (Ochberg, undated). This cycle fosters a sense of deep emotional attachment, and is something that abusers may consciously use to further entrap their victims. Cycles of abuse followed by reward are recognized by torturers the world over as a means of ensuring compliance in victims (Herman, 1992).

## A history of child abuse

Sometimes, women who were sexually, physically or otherwise abused as children come away from these experiences having learned that the people who love them, hurt them. An abusive relationship in which they are further raped and abused may be part of the process of *revictimization,* which may happen when a woman's sense of agency and perception of what love is, are critically damaged by earlier abuse (Herman, 1992). Importantly, this is not an attempt to blame women for further abuse. Rather, it is a necessary acknowledgment of another area of vulnerability that child abuse may leave in its wake, and which abusers may be quick to capitalize upon (Easteal and McOrmond-Plummer, 2006).

## Manipulative abusers

I have referred to manipulative abusers above, and will reiterate here that at the point of losing his partner, a perpetrator may bombard her with positive behaviors aimed primarily at re-establishing control (Bancroft, 2003). A perpetrator may also manipulate his victim's reality, so that she comes to believe that his abusive treatment is her fault, and that it will change if *she* changes. This is true of some IPSV survivors, who may believe that their partners rape them because they are "frigid" or in some other way inadequate. For example, IPSV survivor Charlotte said, "I felt that as long as I stood by Ted, I could help him" (Easteal and McOrmond-Plummer, 2006, p. 111).

### What the victim hears from other people

An abused woman may find that people to whom she turns appear to place a higher priority on her abuser than her safety. She may hear things like, "But he loves you and the kids," "He works so hard for his family," or, "Aren't you glad he's a tiger in the bedroom?" He may actually be a well-liked community member, so she wonders what is wrong with her perception. For example, survivor Nichole said, "He was the type of person everyone loves and I felt that I must love him too" (Easteal & McOrmond-Plummer, 2006, p.112).

### Cognitive dissonance

Cognitive dissonance is the ability to know two opposing things at once, but to suppress knowledge of uncomfortable truths in order to believe something more favorable. This is a known phenomenon with cult members who may have committed hard work, money, and trust to the cult leader, believing that he or she is a savior who loves them and desires the best for them. Then, they may receive evidence that the leader engages in sexual practices that are incongruent with what he or she preaches, and lives a lavish lifestyle on the money and labor of converts who are expected to live in poverty. They may also witness or be subjected to sexual and other abuses by the cult leadership. But cult members who have committed so much expend considerable psychological effort to suppress doubts about the cult and the beloved leader (Baron, 1989). This may also be the case for women who have committed years, love, loyalty and/or children to an abusive partner. They may deny the reality of sexual and other abuse in order to sustain the relationship. Melina, whose child was conceived in a violent rape by her husband, gave an example:

> Years ago when going through the domestic violence proceedings, I was asked if I'd been raped by my husband. I immediately said no, and at the time there's no way I would have recognised it as rape because I was in denial and would have been much too ashamed and afraid of the consequences with my ex-husband. He would have gone totally nuts, I'm sure. I don't want to even guess what that would mean. But stronger than all those feelings is the desire to protect my daughter, for if I was raped by my husband, what does that make my daughter?
>
> (Easteal and McOrmond-Plummer, 2006, p. 110)

### Remember

The above points may be useful in a discussion of factors that help entrap women in relationships of abuse. Exploring these issues with survivors where appropriate may assist them in making informed choices about their lives. However, as we have seen, these points are not the only reasons women profess love for men who have sexually abused them, and they should not be used in condescending or limiting ways to define the experiences of survivors.

## Conclusion

This chapter has attempted to challenge some stereotypes about who rapes, and to examine the reasons why women may love men who sexually assault them. It has hopefully provided insight that will enable professionals, as well as other people who intersect with IPSV survivors and perpetrators, to deliver assistance and justice in a more effective way.

## References

Bancroft, L. (2003). *Why does he do that? Inside the minds of angry and controlling men*. New York, NY: Berkeley Publishing Group.

Baron, R. (1989). *Psychology: The essential science*. Boston, MA: Allyn & Bacon.

Beisner, L. (2014, December 16). An open letter to Dr. Camille Cosby. Role reboot. Retrieved from: www.rolereboot.org/culture-and-politics/details/2014–12-open-letter-dr-camille-cosby/.

Bergen, R. (1996). *Wife rape: Understanding the response of survivors and service providers*. Thousand Oaks, CA: Sage Publications.

CBS Evening News (CBSEveningNews). (2014, December 15). NEW: Billy Cosby's wife Camille releases statement comparing coverage of her husband to Rolling Stone UVA rape story. (Tweet). Retrieved from: https://twitter.com/CBSEveningNews/status/544608377058656256/photo/1.

Cooke, D. (2008, July 18). Wife speaks out on marital sex attacks. *The Sydney Morning Herald*. Retrieved from: www.smh.com.au/national/wife-speaks-out-on-marital-sex-attacks-20080717–3gxj.html.

Easteal, P., & McOrmond-Plummer, L. (2006). *Real rape, real pain: Help for women sexually assaulted by male partners*. Melbourne, Australia: Hybrid Publishers.

Herman, J. (1992). *Trauma and recovery*. New York, NY: Basic Books.

Holmes, R., & Holmes, S. (2002). *Sex crimes: Patterns and behaviour*. Thousand Oaks, CA: Sage Publications.

Matsakis, A. (1996). *I can't get over it: A handbook for trauma survivors*. Oakland, CA: New Harbinger Publications.

Ochberg, F. (n.d.). Understanding the victims of spousal abuse. Retrieved from the Gift from Within website: www.giftfromwithin.org/html/spousal.html.

Russell, D. (1990). *Rape in marriage* (2nd ed.). New York, NY: Macmillan Publishing Company.

Silkstone, D. (2004, February 28). Seeing is not always believing. *The Age*. Retrieved from: www.theage.com.au/articles/2004/02/27/1077676964354.html?from=storyrhs.

# Part 3

# Perpetrators' strategies for control

# Chapter 8

# What intimate partner sexual violence looks like

## Coercive methods of perpetrators

*Louise McOrmond-Plummer*

## Introduction

It is important for professionals who encounter perpetrators (and survivors) to be able to clearly identify the types of behaviors that constitute rape and sexual assault, in order to respond appropriately or confront it in perpetrators. This chapter thus identifies what perpetrators of intimate partner sexual violence (IPSV) may do, and the methods of coercion they frequently use.

## Forms of IPSV

Sexually abusive partners inflict a range of violations, including but not limited to the following:

- Rape, including vaginal, oral or anal penetration. Researchers have commented on the frequent use of anal rape by partners, saying, "In many ways, anal rape appears to be the quintessential way for a man to humiliate his wife" (Finkelhor & Yllo, 1985, p. 30). For other perpetrators, anal rape may be another way of making sure they possess all of the woman, or for the thrill of "breaking in" a different kind of virginity (Russell, 1990, p. 86). Rape may include penetration with finger, penis, or object. Oral rape may include not only forced fellatio, but also cunnilingus.
- Sex acts that have been refused by the survivor in the past.
- Forced sex after giving birth or after surgery – this may be a particularly risky time for IPSV (Bergen, 2006).
- Forcing a partner to watch and/or act out pornography.
- Forcing a partner to have sex in front of others.
- Forced prostitution.
- Sex with animals.
- Sex with other adults or children – this may include setting a partner up for gang rape.
- Forcing a partner to have culturally or religiously taboo sex.
- Degradation during sex.

- Name-calling of a sexual nature in front of others.
- The uploading of intimate photographs of a partner to the Internet, or otherwise passing them around, or threats to do so.
- The gamut of behaviors that may constitute sexual assault, such as forced touching, or forcing the victim to touch the perpetrator.

## A dangerous rising trend: pornography, levels of sadism and physical injury

Di Macleod, director of an Australian sexual assault service, speaks of a large spike in women presenting with serious injuries as a result of sexual assaults by husbands and partners. Much of the violence and injury perpetrated in the course of rape or sexual assault has its roots in the ready availability of online pornography that is becoming more extreme in depicting the eroticization of pain, with the trivializing of rape, and encouragement of lack of empathy. This is the new "sex education" for boys and men, and is impacting in disastrous ways on their future and current partners (Gold Coast Centre Against Sexual Violence, 2016). A British study also reveals a worrying rising trend of coerced and painful anal sex experiences in younger women, which appears to be fueled in part by representations in pornography (Marston & Lewis, 2014). (See Chapter 13 for more on the strong relationship of pornography to much IPSV.)

## Types of coercion in IPSV

Many people still tend to view rape through the lens of social mythology, i.e. it is only rape if it is extremely violent, or if the victim fought sufficiently to "prove" lack of consent, preferably sustaining an injury. While much IPSV does occasion high levels of injury (Myhill & Allen, 2002), many partner rapists also know of ways other than violence to ensure the victim's compliance, rendering sexual acts without consent. For example, one partner rapist says, "I would act like I was mad at her and she would give in. It works every time" (Hite, 1981, p. 776).

Consent is not necessarily the absence of the word "no," and must mean *free agreement* – that is, having the freedom to withdraw consent without facing any negative consequence, either physical or psychological. This is discussed further in Chapter 1.

Relationships are complex, and partners do sometimes agree to sex that they may not really want. Are all such encounters rape? By no means – the determinant factor is whether there is anything to fear as a result of refusal (Anderson, Draughon, & Campbell, 2014). For example, has there been bullying, badgering, or intimidation of any kind, either just before the encounter, or on prior occasions when a partner refused sex? And, if the victim did not say "no," what were the circumstances – for example, was she incapacitated by drugs, or asleep? Will he inform the couple's faith leader about her wifely insubordination? Has he always just "taken" sex in the past, regardless of what she says? There are also ways of withdrawing consent such as tears, just "laying there" or stiffening. If a victim fears she may be beaten, she may even pretend enthusiasm, or may do so to bring a more expedient end to the assault. None of these actions constitutes consent.

It has long been a fixed part of a sexist social structure that boys and men are expected to overcome female resistance to sex by any means necessary. "Coming of age" movies still depict numerous subterfuges that boys may use to "score" – these behaviors are not labeled as rape and sexual assault, but are actively approved as "boys being boys." However, in most Western countries it is now recognized – at least in black-letter law – that submission does not equal consent, as discussed in Chapter 14.

It is also worth remembering that some perpetrators of IPSV do not actually make a show of seeking consent. Some perpetrators deliberately use forced sex to inflict pain on their partner or to assert power over her; these perpetrators *want* the sex to be an *assault* (McOrmond-Plummer, 2014).

Different types of violence or coercion may also suggest different motivations for acts of sexual assault. For a discussion of IPSV perpetrators' motivations specifically, see Chapter 4.

Let us now turn our attention to methods of coercion. Please note that there are a number of ways that a victim's consent may be negated that do not fall under the following categories. These include: depriving her of liberty, for example entrapment in a room; refusal to allow her to tend to children; and raping her when she is incapacitated by drugs or alcohol, or asleep.

### Emotional coercion

As indicated above, not all IPSV contains elements of additional physical violence. The threats used in emotional coercion are generally of a nonviolent nature, but may nevertheless be extremely distressing (Russell, 1990).

The following are some types of emotional coercion that Easteal and McOrmond-Plummer (2006) identified as having taken place for women in their sample:

- A teenage boy says he will "dump" his girlfriend, or spread rumors about her if she does not agree to sex with him.
- A husband quotes scripture to manipulate his wife into sex.
- A woman's partner threatens to seek sexual satisfaction elsewhere.
- Repeated badgering for a partner to engage in sexual practices she has stated she does not like.
- Treating a partner coldly for refusing sex.
- Treating children poorly because their mother refused sex.
- Refusing to permit a partner to sleep until she gives in to a sexual demand.

With respect to impact on the victim, rape and sexual assault by emotional coercion do result in harm to the victim. Research using the Trauma Symptoms Inventory reveals that women who have experienced this type of coercion score more similarly to women who have experienced rape or attempted rape, than to women who have experienced no victimization (Broach & Peretric, 2006). Further, Russell's (1990) study found that, while 70% of IPSV survivors interviewed said they were "extremely upset" by threats of a physical nature, a larger proportion of the women (83%) were "extremely upset" by a partner's threats to leave or withdraw his love.

Sex after capitalizing on a partner's insecurities or fears to get her to acquiesce is rape. This contradicts the views of some in the community that women should be "big" enough to deal with this, and not go "crying rape" (Easteal and McOrmond-Plummer, 2006). Once again, we see focus on what the victim does or does not do to avoid rape, rather than how her partner is abdicating his responsibility to respect her right to withdraw consent. This also fails to account for entrenched dynamics in abusive relationships, wherein a woman's sense of rights and autonomy may be completely worn down.

And, with respect to women who do dig their heels in and say no, emotional coercion may also proceed physical force. For example, a man may unsuccessfully verbally badger his partner for sex and then roll her over and do it anyway (Easteal & McOrmond-Plummer, 2006). The crucial factor is that "no" means "no," however it is expressed.

### Threats to a third party

While this sort of verbal threat resembles the verbal coercion described above, the threats here are typically of a more physical nature. A perpetrator may threaten harm to his partner's children, friends, family, workmates, or pets if she doesn't do what he wants sexually. For example, Summer, an IPSV survivor, says, "I was told if I didn't give him the blowjob the way he wanted it that he would have my daughter do it for him once he left" (Easteal & McOrmond-Plummer, 2006, p. 70). These threats may also involve damaging or destroying property the victim values. Such threats may be terrifying, especially when a woman knows her partner is fully capable of making good on them.

### Threats of harm to the victim

A perpetrator can enforce sexual compliance by threatening to beat, kill, or otherwise harm his partner. He may threaten to have her raped by others. Or, he may threaten a certain type of rape if she does not acquiesce to another, i.e. that he will anally rape her if she does not submit to vaginal sex, and he may set up scenarios in which he makes her "choose" the way she is raped (Easteal & McOrmond-Plummer, 2006).

The threat of harm may be either explicit or implicit when a perpetrator has just beaten his partner, and – as IPSV perpetrators frequently do – demands sex in the aftermath. Women understand that refusal will result in further beatings, and that they will be raped anyway, only more violently than if they simply submit. Courts unfortunately do not always recognize that historical physical violence in a relationship may be a factor in intimidation of IPSV victims, negating their consent (Carline & Easteal, 2014).

The use of weapons to force acquiescence to sex is also a clear and credible threat of harm to the victim. As I was researching for my first book some 15 years ago, I had a moving letter from a woman in her eighties, who spoke of how her late husband had always "put [sexual] rebellion down with a gun" (private communication, McOrmond-Plummer, 2001). Such a threat may also be implicit; for example, Anderson, Draughon, and Campbell (2014) wrote about a woman who never refused sex because she knew that her husband kept a gun beneath the bed – and he knew that she knew.

### Physical force

Physically forcing a partner into sex may include:

- Beating her into submission, or engaging in acts that hurt her.
- Restraints such as ropes or handcuffs, or pinioning her arms.
- Strangulation.
- Using physical strength to hold her down or lie on top of her.
- Knocking her unconscious or deliberately rendering her unconscious with drugs or alcohol.

*An important note about forcible rape with additional physical violence, threats of physical violence, or the use of weapons*: Anderson, Draughon, and Campbell (2014, p. 61) write, "Although it is important for providers to be aware of sexually coercive acts which can result in mental health sequelae such as PTSD, it is physically forced sex which is a risk factor for intimate partner homicide." This makes it essential to understand that rape occurring in physically violent relationships, or that in itself occasions additional violence or threats of violence, is a red flag for potential fatality to the woman. Domestic violence advocates, police and other key players must assess for physically forced sex, and take steps to ensure that the woman is protected from the perpetrator accordingly. (See Chapter 2 for more about IPSV as a fatality risk in domestic violence.)

### Conclusion

This chapter has been written to give a brief overview of perpetrator behaviors that may constitute or facilitate IPSV. This knowledge is particularly important for those who work with perpetrators, or who may subscribe to myths about what IPSV is. Recognition is a crucial part of ensuring that these crimes do not continue to flourish in an environment of ignorance about them, and that women are made safer.

## References

Anderson, J., Draughon, J., & Campbell, J. (2014). Fatality and health risks associated with intimate partner sexual violence. In L. McOrmond-Plummer, P. Easteal, & J.Y. Levy-Peck (Eds.), *Intimate partner sexual violence: A multidisciplinary guide to improving services and support for survivors of rape and abuse* (pp. 54–64). London, UK: Jessica Kingsley Publishers.

Bergen, R.K. (2006). Marital rape: New research and directions. Retrieved from: www.vawnet.org/research/summary.php?doc_id=248&find_type=web_desc_AR.

Broach, J.L., & Peretric, P.A. (2006). Beyond traditional definitions of assault: Expanding our focus to include sexually coercive experiences. *Journal of Family Violence, 21*(8), 477–468.

Carline, A., & Easteal P. (2014). *Shades of grey: Domestic and sexual violence against women: Law reform and society.* London, UK: Routledge.

Easteal, P., & McOrmond-Plummer, L. (2006). *Real rape, real pain: Help for women sexually abused by male partners.* Melbourne, Australia: Hybrid Press.

Finkelhor, D., & Yllo, K. (1985). *License to rape: Sexual abuse of wives.* New York, NY: The Free Press.

Gold Coast Centre of Sexual Violence, Inc. (2016). Submission to Parliament of Australia, Environment and Communications References Committee – Inquiry into the harm being done to Australian children through access to pornography on the Internet. Unpublished manuscript.

Hite, S. (1981). *The Hite Report on male sexuality: How men feel about love, sex, and relationships.* New York, NY: Knopf/Random House.

McOrmond-Plummer, L. (2014). Preventing secondary wounding by misconception: What professionals really need to know about intimate partner sexual violence. In L. McOrmond-Plummer, P. Easteal, & J.Y. Levy-Peck (Eds.), *Intimate partner sexual violence: A multidisciplinary guide to improving services and support for survivors of rape and abuse.* London, UK: Jessica Kingsley Publishers.

Marston, C., & Lewis, R. (2014). Anal heterosex among young people and implications for health promotion: A qualitative study in the UK. *BMJ Open, 4*(8), e004996-e004996. http://dx.doi.org/10.1136/bmjopen-2014-004996.

Myhill, A., & Allen, J. (2002). Rape and sexual assault of women: Findings from the British Crime Survey. Retrieved from: www.aphroditewounded.org/Myhill and Allen.pdf.

Russell, D. (1990). *Rape in marriage.* Bloomington, IN: Indiana University Press.

# Chapter 9

# "But he didn't hit me!"*
## Living with a non-physical-battering sexual abuser

*Lindsey Mason*

## Context

We both belonged to a fundamentalist church, which was patriarchal in its belief systems. I had been brought up in the church; my husband's family had joined when Craig was a teenager. We first met in the UK at a youth study week organized and run by the church. At the time I was just 16 and he had just turned 26. I thought he was immature and paid little notice of him.

The second time we met was about a year later, at a Bible school. I had invited a mutual friend, Tim, who had told me he was bringing a friend who was depressed and he thought the week might benefit him. During the long bus ride down to the Alps, Tim persuaded me to go and sit next to Craig as he was feeling depressed and isolated, and asked me to simply chat with him to cheer him up a bit. I was not a particularly sociable person, but kind-hearted, and Craig and I spent a number of hours chatting during that coach trip. As the week progressed, we spent more and more time together. I did notice that Craig seemed to take a dislike to any other lad whom I also spent time with. During that week, Craig asked me to accompany him on a walk and confided in me that as a younger teen, he had at one point sexually touched a girl when riding past her on his bike. I felt as though I could have fainted, knocked over by a feather, but continued to listen to him.

Craig explained that at the time he was very confused about the difference between love and sex, and was generally in a mess emotionally (he had learning difficulties and had been put in a special school where there were only two options: either you were bullied or you were a bully, and he had chosen the latter). He seemed truly remorseful of his previous behavior and had since been baptized (wiping away all previous sins). He also told me that when he had confided the same story in his last girlfriend, she had simply ended the relationship immediately. This had left him feeling even worse about himself and he doubted that any girl or woman would ever trust him enough to go out with him. Despite my own inclination to run, I carried on walking and chatting with him. There was no overt flirting or insinuation that we were a couple or even heading that way. I was very academic and studied Scripture avidly; we talked about biblical issues and the forgiveness of sins.

Within a week of returning from that Bible school, I received a letter from Craig, in which he declared that I had made him so happy that he could think of nothing else but me. This letter was almost like a love letter, and again, I was completely taken aback. I did not know how to respond. The last thing I had intended was to flirt or encourage him in any way to think of me as a potential girlfriend, and yet somehow it seemed to me that I must have given him exactly that message. He considered me a gift from God.

My parents had recently separated and I felt I could not talk to them. Going to anyone outside of the church for advice was also frowned upon, so I responded, trying to encourage Craig in biblical studies or talking of other things such as my hobbies. This carried on for a few months, with letters flying to and fro. One of Craig's closest friends said that he was very concerned about Craig, that if I were to break up this relationship (!?) as the previous girlfriend had done, then he believed seriously that Craig would commit suicide. This hit me hard, as only a few months beforehand, I had lost a friend to suicide. I became Craig's girlfriend, though we sort of drifted in more out of his assumption that we were an item rather than any real discussion or decision on the matter.

In our church, sex before marriage was a complete no-no. I, as a female, was under the authority of my father until I was married and then the authority over me was automatically passed on to my husband. Marriage itself was the joining sexually together – that was marriage in God's eyes, and should not occur before the wedding. Petting was permitted to an extent, which most young couples probably took to extremes but refrained from going all the way. I have no recollection of specifically discussing this with Craig. I just assumed that his beliefs were the same as mine, as we belonged to the same church and would have been taught the same beliefs and values.

While I was outwardly going along with the relationship (long-distance, since we lived in separate countries), I was inwardly hoping that once I got to university, the relationship would just gradually fall apart. I was headed toward Oxford, my application already accepted and the grades they were asking were easy for me to fulfil. Craig, on the other hand, had left the special school with no qualification and was working as a kitchen hand – there was a huge gulf not only in our education and social standing, but also in our intellectual abilities and hopes for the future.

## The first sexual assault and early marriage

One night, when I was visiting Craig at his parent's house (where he still lived), we were petting pretty heavily, and suddenly, he simply went all the way. There was no prior talk about it, no condom, no requesting of consent. I cannot even remember whether I asked him what he was doing or to stop. He just inserted his penis into my vagina, came and rolled over. I was stunned. It had never occurred to me that he would even consider going all the way, because of our beliefs. In those few minutes, he had made me his wife. In God's sight, we were married and from then on, he referred to me in private as his wife. With that one act, my life was no longer my own, but his. I now recognize this as a form of marriage by rape, but at the time I did not know it was rape. I was 18, still at school, and trapped.

From then on there was no point in holding back, so sex occurred regularly. I would try to persuade him to wear condoms, but he would take them off half-way through intercourse or refuse outright, because it spoiled his pleasure. I believe now he was also keen for me to get pregnant. He began pressuring me not to go to university, because he was concerned that it would increase the educational gulf between us and could be a cause of stress in our marriage, so I cancelled my place at Oxford. Craig asked my father for permission to marry me, and my father, although initially against the relationship, agreed.

Shortly after I finished my final exams, my father found out that we had been having sex, and threw me out of the house for committing such a sin. I had nowhere to go but to Craig and his family. So in the middle of 1992 I set off for the UK. By the end of that year we were married. I walked down the aisle and said my vows with the full intention of being the good Christian wife Craig wanted and needed. My obligation now was to him, to fulfil his needs, wishes and dreams.

Prior to marriage, Craig had been very keen to have sex and spend as much time with me as possible. Once we were married this changed. We moved into a small flat above a shop which closed with security shutters at 5:30 pm each day. I was physically unable to open the shutters, so had to ensure I was at home before the shop closed. Most evenings, Craig would return home late, having had dinner with his parents (though before we married, he had not a good word to say about his mother), even though I always had an evening meal prepared for him. His desire for sex lessened, though he was keen to start a family as soon as possible. He also did not want me to meet up with other men as he was so insecure, so I limited any and all interaction with men. Every weekend was spent with his parents and the church members.

## Moving to Switzerland

I had my first child when I was 21 and by 26 I had four children under five, two of whom had obvious learning difficulties. During the same time, we had moved house five times. When we found out the third baby was on its way, my father suggested we return to Switzerland, since we would be financially better off there. I was keen on moving "back home" but adamant that the decision had to lie with my husband, as it was a foreign country to him and he would be leaving his family behind. But Craig was equally adamant that it would be in the best interest of all to move to Switzerland, not least because he felt he was still attached to his mother's apron strings and believed the distance would help break that bond.

I was happy in Switzerland – for the first time in our marriage. I no longer felt isolated and depressed. My daughter with learning difficulties could have the assessments and therapies needed and my eldest was attending a preschool group he adored. Initially, Craig also made efforts to learn German and found work, but his tendency of not cooperating well in groups and finding fault with each boss and employee led to him being fired from two consecutive jobs. He returned to the UK, supposedly just temporarily to earn some money, but promised he would stay in touch regularly. He didn't. I would phone him and plead for him to at least speak with the children and with me and to return home just once every six weeks for a few days, often only hearing him swearing about me before coming to the phone.

A few months later, Craig informed me casually that he had decided to return to the UK regardless of whether the children and I accompanied him back. He had already told his family about this decision. I was devastated. For the first time we had no financial troubles, I was able to mother my children, and the children were getting the help and treatment they needed. I was shocked at his selfishness – he was considering what *he* wanted, rather than what was in the best interest of the family. I told him I was completely against that decision but would return with him to keep the family together, even though I knew I was returning to poverty, isolation and a general lack of support, both for myself and the children. Only a week later I found I was expecting my fourth child.

We returned to the UK and Craig started working for himself, and I was left basically to act as a single parent, but with the added burden of acting as his receptionist, accountant, and cleaner for the business. Even so, financially we were again in a mess, so I also sought work I could do from home. I had to remain home just in case a call came through for him.

Again, Craig would often not return home until all the children were in bed, preferring to spend the evening with his parents. Any marital difficulties he considered we had, he would discuss with his parents, mainly his mother, and then she would come round to me and give me an earful about what a dreadful wife I was. I would have to beg my husband to set the matter straight. He would cause the upset, but then he would be the savior who reconciled us again. Emotionally, he was my prosecutor and defender. This pattern of triangulation continued well beyond the marriage and to this day.

It was also while expecting our fourth child, that I first found pornography in his van. His use of pornography increased as the sexual violence toward me did. He told me that while I was gross due to being pregnant; these images reminded him of me when I was not pregnant. While I was pregnant, Craig would not want to touch my tummy, saying it felt as though I had an alien or monster in me. He hated the change in my body shape, except my enlarged breasts. When breastfeeding, he was almost jealous of the baby who could touch my breasts any time, but got moody with me if I asked him not to touch them in bed because the nipples were sore. He was also largely uninterested in the children unless someone else was present, when he played "dad of the week."

## The second stage of sexual assaults: buggery (anal rape)

By the time the last baby was about six months old, I started reverting to some of my former independence. I started reading more, wanted to take courses to increase my qualifications and have better job prospects too. We argued a lot about these things. I began to recognize that there were aspects of my husband's behavior which I could not control or change by discussion, so instead I would avoid the issue.

It was around that time that the second stage of sexual abuse began: buggery. Again, one night he just buggered me instead of having normal intercourse. There was no discussion about it beforehand, and he had never been keen on experimenting in bed before and most definitely not on me initiating anything. I thought it was a mistake, but he made it clear in the morning that it was no mistake, that he enjoyed this "new" way of doing things. And that is how it carried on with me tolerating being buggered more and more frequently, and trying to discuss with him how it made me feel and the health effects it was having on me. But I never really said *"no,"* I will *not* agree to being buggered – though I tried to indicate it in other ways. And he never asked either verbally or by his actions, confirmed whether I was giving my consent: for about two-and-a-half years it was simply tolerated.

## The effects of tolerating buggery

Years and years of buggery. I tolerated it. In that sense it was with consent. A nice term which negates all the subterfuge, the manipulating which goes on. Guilt, confusion, hope. Guilt at not being physically "good enough." After four kids I was loose, or so he said. Doing things normally wasn't exciting any more. This was new, interesting, exciting. He looked forward to it. Drove round in his van and looked forward to it, even after it was definitely without consent, when it was rape. So I felt guilty about not being good enough, for being unhappy about something he obviously enjoyed. And confused. I told him, told him time and time again, please not so often, please not tonight, please do it normally. I explained that it was not comfortable, that it hurt sometimes, that I got terrible tummy cramps the following day, and diarrhea, and piles. I asked him just not to do it so often. I can't remember it making any difference. It would go on, often two, three, four times a week. He would say he enjoyed it. Did I? How did I feel about it? I would explain that the build-up was enjoyable, but I got nothing from the act itself, and was then left without satisfaction and only tummy-ache and piles the next day. To me, that should have been enough for him to at least reduce the frequency, but it didn't. I never could understand that. That is what I mean about confusion, I had explained to him that the act itself did nothing for me sexually, emotionally, and that physically it had awful side-effects. And it never changed his actions toward me. His preference and pleasure came before concern for me.

There was one time I remember because I was so surprised. He was buggering me and it was really hurting. Finally I cried out and said, "Stop, please, stop, that hurts." And he did. He turned me over and raped me instead. I was grateful for that.

Finally, I simply could not stand it any longer. I had taken more abuse than I thought I could bear. I had a really nasty nipple infection, due to being mauled by dirty hands. It was so bad, it looked as though there was a hole in the nipple and it was going to fall off. I showed him. That might seem like an odd thing to do, show your nipples to someone who is raping you on a regular basis. But I knew how squeamish he was about such things, and it meant that he didn't touch them from then on. And that was relief in itself. At least he wasn't touching my breasts – a little bit more of me that wasn't taken.

When asked once, was the anal sex with consent, I said that I had tolerated it. How little that says. To tolerate something that is done with some form of consent simply doesn't explain the confusion, the emotional pressure to try to comply, to try to please, even pressure to enjoy or maintain that I enjoyed it, when it was perfectly obvious that I didn't. I became, even in my own mind, simply something/one who was there so he could have some enjoyment, not a person with feelings or any rights over her body. That made 100% rape possible. In both our minds I had no right to say no, and he no responsibility to take my feelings into account.

## The final stages of sexual abuse: The official rapes

We spent the Christmas holidays 2000 in Switzerland. I had been getting more and more depressed and confused about my feelings and responsibilities toward Craig. I told him that I was really struggling with all the buggery and his lack of addressing my concerns around it or taking my feelings and health into consideration, and generally struggling and feeling confused about any bedroom activity, that I was falling into severe depression and also felt happier in the company of other male friends than with him, which to me was a warning sign that we needed to redress the balance in our marriage. I asked for time out sexually to try to get my head straight and to work out what I was feeling. Craig agreed to my having time out from all sexual activity starting immediately. We returned to my dad's house, did the daily Bible readings and prayer together, then went to bed. That night Craig raped me – twice. I cannot remember whether it was anal or vaginal, whether he said anything or not, I cannot remember any details at all, just know that it happened and that it was such a shock to me that I froze completely (no fight or flight response: as with all the other assaults, I was like a rabbit in the headlights). Over the next three months, I counted over 70 sexual assaults, all including anal and/or vaginal penetration.

At the beginning of the fourth month, we sat down on a Sunday afternoon, and discussed the whole thing again. I simply could not cope with having to go to bed each night and either being raped or waiting to be raped. I needed at the very least to be able to have the occasional night when I was safe. He explained that his sex-drive was extremely high. He didn't quite understand why, because throughout the marriage it had been sporadic and, if anything, low. I still wanted to find some way of sorting this whole thing out, so I suggested we reach an agreement which would stop the rapes. If, on the majority of nights, I agreed to intercourse, then he would respect and honor my saying no on the other nights. I had to come up with some sort of solution because he denied any ability to control himself. He agreed.

That night, Sunday, I said "No, I am tired," and he honored it. That gave me hope.

Monday, I said "Yes," feeling I had to make the effort to respond. That was so difficult. But I had to show I was willing to try.

Tuesday, I again gave my consent. I felt under a lot of pressure to say yes, that I felt I had no option but to give consent. I know it felt as though I was being raped but even more confusing. I was disgusted at myself. It felt as though I had agreed to be raped.

Wednesday, I was working during the evening. I got back tired and as I got into bed I told him no, not tonight, I was tired. He said I couldn't do that; it wasn't fair. I had to let him know earlier on in the evening because he had been looking forward to it all evening. And he raped me anyway. I was completely devastated. The agreement had failed. There was no negotiating, no safety for even one night. I had tried to buy myself a few nights without being assaulted and humiliated, and he had denied me even that. Total despair. There seemed no way to end it, no way of escape, no getting through to him. No hope.

## Doubts creep in . . . and trying to avoid being assaulted

I honestly believed him when he told me he could not control himself, that he didn't want to do it, but it was some sort of compulsion which he struggled against in vain. I wanted to believe him, as the alternative was that he was purposely raping me. I had to believe him to maintain some hope that we could get over these problems and that it would stop.

I remember the day that I first doubted him. During a discussion he mentioned that he looked forward to it, while driving around all day. That sickened me. How can you look forward to raping someone? And that didn't tally with what he had said on so many occasions – namely, that he would try to stop himself but couldn't, that he would be convinced and determined not to touch me until I got into bed, and then he couldn't help himself. On another occasion he said he looked forward to it all evening, got really excited about it. I knew then that he could control it but he chose not to. He chose to rape me. It just took a while to sink in.

For a long time I actually believed he was sexually assaulting me against his will. I interpreted his threats as statements of fact that he could not control. I bought in to his justifications, his blame-shifting, his denial of responsibility. I wanted to believe him, wanted to believe well of him. I wanted to believe it was me causing the abuse, because then I had the power to stop it. I had choice: I just had to find the right formula. I believed I was constantly causing him to sin by being there because he couldn't help it.

When I moved into the Refuge (domestic violence shelter), it was with him in mind as much as myself. It was to stop the downward spiral. To give me a breather, and to remove myself from him, to stop him sinning. My hope was that by stopping the downward spiral and putting some distance between us, we would be able to sort it all out better. It was meant to be temporary, until I could come home again.

It was nearly ten weeks once he had gone before I returned home to stay. I had asked a solicitor to write him a formal letter due to his assaults on me, but also because there was bruising on my daughter and both the girls said Daddy had done it. When I asked him, he said they were both lying to cause trouble for him.

And they say: marital rape is not as bad as stranger rape. I don't know. I have never been raped by a stranger. But I think being raped by your husband in your own home must be worse in some ways. When it is the person you have entrusted your life to who abuses you, it isn't just physical or sexual assault, it is a betrayal of the very core of your marriage, or your person, your trust. If you are not safe in your own home, next to your husband, where are you safe?

## Buggery and force-only rape: the reality and the consequences

During the time I realized I was being raped, the buggery was preferable. It was less personal, and he was less likely to try kissing me. When you are being raped on such a frequent basis you hold on to the little things. You count your blessings. And any further violation is terrifying. Like when he tried sucking my nipples and I tried to move his head off, so he grabbed both my arms and flung them above my head, held them there and continued sucking my breasts and nipples. That was a really horrible one, which sticks out in my mind, and still makes me feel physically sick. Not only did he rape me, but he had taken another step, had touched me intimately with his mouth, and had displayed enough force or violence actually (he always used force to hold me exactly where he wanted me) to ensure I couldn't fight him off again. He held my arms by the wrists with one of his hands and held them so tight and with so much of his weight on them, that they really hurt and then started losing any sensation.

When he finally let go I did not make the same mistake again. I simply laid them next to my body, pressed up against my sides; even though he was all over my front, he was not getting near my sides. I remember trying to avoid his mouth by moving my head from side to side. Didn't work of course, simply held my head where he wanted it when he got fed up of my thrashing it around. Revolting. Grotesque.

It is the waiting I remember most. Waiting for him to return at night, shaking like a leaf, feeling sick, smoking like a trooper. Being the last to leave, trying to put off coming home. Stopping halfway for a cigarette, trying to compose myself and gather strength and courage to go back. Waiting downstairs, reading or listening to music until the early hours of the morning, hoping that he would be really sound asleep before I got to bed. I would try to get into bed really, really quietly and slowly so as not to wake him. Ensure I didn't touch him, and curl up right up against the wall, hardly daring to breathe. It never did work; he woke.

## The normal pattern for rapes and assaults

I remember the feeling when he turned toward me in bed and put his hand on my side. I would be filled with a surge of fear, panic. It was like a death-toll. I would plead with him, beg him, try to move away or get up, try moving his hand, try to reason with him. It never made any difference. Once his hand was there it would not move away. I don't remember any response from him verbally apart from the initial "It'll be fun," "Come on, you'll enjoy it," or the "You would do it for Bobby." Toward the middle of the four-and-a-half months, if not earlier, there was no response, no talk. Just this hand. Firmly holding me in place, not possible to budge. And then it would start to move up, slowly, decidedly, while the other hand continued to hold me. I would be rigid, my arms crossed tightly across my breasts, trying to stop that hand. But he is so much stronger than I am. He would easily push my arms out of the way and maul my breasts, squeezing, pulling, pinching, rubbing, all so hard it would hurt. He would pull my pants down. Off for rape; to the knees for buggery. No amount of trying to wriggle or squirm would help. I would just be held tighter and forced down on his penis. That would hurt. From that point on there is nothing in most cases. Most assaults have rolled into one, always following the same pattern. I don't remember feeling anything either physically or emotionally most of the time. It was as though my mind and my body became disconnected during the assaults. I guess that is another form of dissociation, a coping or survival mechanism built into our system which enables us to cope with the "uncopable." Then it would be over. He would come, he always did. He simply turned over and went to sleep.

And in the morning, he would bring me up a cup of tea. As though nothing had happened.

Confusion features very high on the list of feelings I remember experiencing at that time. Like the time he stripped me naked and raped me, having picked me up by my breasts from behind and dragged/carried me to the settee. Afterward, he made me a cup of coffee, then sat down next to me to drink his, as though we had just made love. That sort of thing is so damn confusing. I knew he had just raped me, stripped me forcefully and held me down. It was too awful to accept. And here he was, acting as though nothing abnormal had happened.

I lied to people. I didn't tell anyone for months about that incident. The police called for weeks, encouraging me to charge him for the rapes and buggery. And I could not tell them it was still going on. I remember they called and asked whether he had assaulted me again. I said no, it was okay at the moment.

## Who was responsible?

I felt responsible for his behavior toward me. He made it perfectly clear that it was my fault, that he couldn't control this urge. I remember him telling me that he went to bed determined not to rape me, but that when I came to bed he just couldn't stop it. He seemed genuinely upset about this. I completely bought into that fallacy and felt sorry for him, poor chap, who desperately didn't want to hurt me but could not stop himself. I actually remember him saying that if I didn't say no, that it wouldn't happen. I guess that makes some sort of sense, if consent is not withheld, then intercourse without consent cannot take place. But the result of that statement and many more like it was that I felt responsible for his sexual abuse of me. It was me causing the rape and buggery by objecting to it. And since I really believed it was my fault, then surely I could also stop it somehow.

## Living with a sexually and emotionally abusive man

He was very intimidating at times, and there were several times I was scared stiff. I remember when he smashed the chair in the kitchen. It was a Sunday afternoon and I was making dinner. It was quite warm and the children were playing outside. He had said it wasn't really rape; "Rape is when you are grabbed by a stranger in a dark alley and raped." I said, "Rape by your husband is worse, because it is in your own home and by a person you love and trust." He didn't like that. He was halfway through a very loud, angry retort when our daughter walked into the kitchen. He picked up a wooden chair and brought it down on the floor so hard it crumbled under his hands. I ushered my little girl out, reassured her and made sure all the kids were out of earshot. Inside he was tearing the rest of the chair apart with bare hands.

He used to regularly hit things when I confronted him about his behavior: the settee, chair, walls, dishwasher, table, etc. I especially remember the dishwasher, because I had my feet on the dishwasher at the time. Again, I had dared to disagree with him on something. He brought both fists down on the dish-washer within inches of my foot so hard it seemed to bounce and rattled. I was scared. It made me jump. The message was clear enough – that could be you. It was not only a display of anger; it was intimidation. I remember he looked at me and said he really felt like hitting me, but that he wouldn't, because then I would have something to show and I would love that. I didn't push it any further.

Even when he left, I knew he was sure I would fold within a few weeks, would not be able to survive without him, and would be on my knees begging him to return. He had told me as much on so many occasions: "You would be lost without me," "If I cannot rape you, then I will rape someone else and it will be your fault," etc. He had done his best to ensure I break down. Quite apart from all the abuse, he had invested a lot of time and effort into demolishing my support base.

Surviving is a strange thing. I am a survivor of emotional and sexual abuse. It sounds so neat, so final. But I don't know that it is ever final. Maybe we are simply in a state of surviving every day. So many things are still a struggle. Going to bed, getting up, leaving the house, talking to anyone, collecting the kids from school, going to work, phoning someone, doing anything. Some days I am frightened of my own shadow; everything presents danger, I cannot stop shaking, am haunted by constant flashbacks, can't eat properly, smoke like a chimney, repeat actions, words, sentences over and over in my head. Other days I am basically all right. And physically it has also left a mark – repeat urinary tract infections, sore nipples, and the scars are still on my face.

## Conclusion

Daily life with a non-physical battering sexual abuser was in many ways similar to that experienced by any domestic violence victim. I was isolated from friends and family due to his insecurities, not permitted outside activities which would allow me to compare my experiences to those of others, I was under his constant and direct control, he ensured we were penniless (financial abuse), and moved us repeatedly so that no social contacts could be grown. The sexual abuse was confusing and has done long-term damage, but the emotional abuse and threats, were and remain far more demobilizing – 16 years after walking away from the marriage, I still show every symptom of PTSD – and *still* have to deal with Craig as a co-parent who not only counters everything I try to do with the children, but still keeps me isolated by blaming me for the marriage breakup and bad-mouthing me to people, including my own children and family. He is still making me pay as he believes himself to be the victim in this story.

## Editors' note

★ This chapter, which was written by a survivor of intimate partner sexual violence (IPSV), is included for its clear depiction of the tactics and behavior of a perpetrator and the dynamics of IPSV. All names except that of the author, and other potential identifiers have been changed.

Readers versed in the dynamics of domestic violence will recognize several manifestations of coercive control in Craig's behavior, such as financial abuse, jealousy, suppression of his partner's independence, and acting out violence on objects as a way of issuing physical threats. Certainly, Craig appears to have subscribed to dangerous patriarchal notions of a woman's place, and of sexual entitlement.

With respect to IPSV, Lindsey's story reveals how many perpetrators know of, and use, other powerful means instead of physical violence to coerce their partners into unwanted sexual contact. Note that spiritual abuse – the misuse of scriptural concepts in order to coerce sex – was a prominent feature of Craig's rapes of Lindsey. In writing of marital rape, Finkelhor and Yllo (1985) refer to methods of coercion that play on deeply entrenched notions of "wifely duty" as *social coercion* (pp. 86–87).

And while the author of this chapter, like many survivors of IPSV, was confused about whether she "consented" to Craig's demands in order to avoid being forcefully raped, and thus drew a distinction between "official" and "un-official" rape, Lindsey was in fact forced into a position of nonchoice, and had to submit to sex acts she did not like in order to avoid being forced. When a woman submits to sex because there is a present threat, she *is* being raped. Readers will note that Craig seemed happy for his wife to blame herself for the rapes, believing as she once did that they were the outcome of nonconsent.

This brings us to the methods that perpetrators of IPSV may use in order to avoid responsibility and consequences (Easteal and McOrmond-Plummer, 2006). With Craig, we see:

- Denial: i.e. Craig tells Lindsey that "rape is when it's a stranger in an alleyway," and at other times behaves as if nothing out of the ordinary had occurred.
- Blame: According to Craig, doing things "normally" is no longer exciting as Lindsey's vagina is loose from multiple childbirths.
- Claiming loss of control: Craig attempts to convince Lindsey that he doesn't want to rape her and even attempts not to do so, but ultimately cannot help himself.

In their three types of marital rape, Finkehor and Yllo (1985, p. 50) write of "obsessive rape." This refers to the partner rapist whose arousal appears to be fueled by specific perverse acts he forces or coerces his partner to engage in. The acts may have a bizarre, ritualistic quality. He may use pornography, and write, talk or think obsessively about specific sex acts. It does not matter to him that his partner does not share his predilections; he is prepared to force them on her. He is not concerned that the acts may cause his partner pain or even, as in Lindsey's case, physical illness. Craig's behavior – his use of pornography combined with his admission of driving around all day looking forward to anally raping his wife, and finally his lack of empathy for her emotional and physical pain – seems to fit the obsessive typology.

Perpetrators must be held accountable for the full effects of their crimes. It is thus important to note that even without the adjunct of physical battery, Lindsey' self-reported trauma has been extensive and long-lasting.

## References

Easteal, P., & McOrmond-Plummer, L. (2006). *Real rape, real pain: Help for women sexually assaulted by male partners*. Melbourne, Australia: Hybrid Press.

Finkelhor, D., & Yllo, K. (1985). *License to rape: Sexual abuse of wives*. New York, NY: The Free Press.

# Chapter 10

# Lucky to be alive
## A battering partner rapist

*Louise McOrmond-Plummer*

## Introduction

I was a single mother aged 18, living in a flat with my beautiful son and nurturing the dream of furthering my education one day, when a neighbor introduced me to a man we'll call Richard. He seemed nice, but I was dating a few men and did not want to be in a steady relationship. I was not initially attracted to him, but we became friends. We had long talks over coffee. I felt for him because he seemed to have had a hard life. He could also be very funny. The attraction developed, and we became a couple.

Richard wanted me to sleep with him, but I wanted to wait. He was offended and angry that I would not trust him sexually. He swore indignantly that he would never do anything to hurt me, and resented the implications of my making him wait. Richard told me that sex would be another expression of his love for me.

Physical and sexual violence did not commence until after we had sex. Lundy Bancroft (2003, p. 175) writes that commencement of sex may be a catalyst for abuse when an abuser thinks, "I have power over you because we have sex." It certainly seemed as if having had sex with Richard granted him a sense of ownership. The abuse escalated quickly, and I blamed myself for letting down my guard. Because I was aware that unmarried mothers are often viewed as less worthy of respect than other women, I had been very cautious about the intentions of men. Richard had known I was vulnerable to the fear of being treated badly, and he took perverse pleasure in using that against me.

The red flags that have been identified for domestic violence (Wilson, 1997) were present: jealousy and possessiveness, crude and demeaning attitudes toward women, quick involvement, and many more. However, like many women, I did not recognize the warning signs. And there were still the good times. However, within two years, I had been beaten and raped more times than I could count. I was lucky to escape with an additional child and my life.

I have learned that what was happening to me was not unusual; in some ways, Richard was a fairly typical batterer. And yet there is still a large gulf in wider society between the understanding that some men *beat* their partners, and understanding that these same men often also *rape* their partners. To bridge the gulf, this chapter will give prominence to the sexual abuse I experienced, with physical abuse as a backdrop.

Partner rape gets lost all too often under the heading of battery, but if we are to effect change, we must not shy away from calling men like Richard *rapists* as well as batterers. I wrote elsewhere about how sexual violence may differ from physical violence: "In my experience, the battery was aimed at getting me to do what I was told or hurting me for not doing so, but the rape had a far nastier and more contemptuous message. It was more calculated to inflict psychological harm than the battery" (McOrmond-Plummer, 2014, p. 46). As much as possible, what you will read below will be about *Richard* – the things he did and how I have come to understand them, based on the passage of time and on the enlightening research of others. Emma Williamson (2014) writes that it is concerning when sexual violence in abusive relationships is considered in isolation rather than as an ongoing and systematic pattern of abuse. Richard did indeed use sexual violence in a systematic way, with certain outcomes in mind. I trust that this will be evident to readers also, and it is especially important for professionals to note.

## Triggers for rape

Below are some common triggers that, in my experience, led to sexual assault/ rape. Readers may note that the sexual assaults I describe were generally employed by Richard to achieve aims that were *not* sexual; sometimes he did not even ejaculate. The message conveyed was more important. This is crucial to know because many people are inclined to confuse IPSV with "sex," rather than the act of violence, control, and degradation that it is. Also, while I have separated triggers into subheadings for clarity, an overlap of purpose may sometimes be noted – for example, rape motivated by jealousy may also be about exerting control.

### Quelling defiance

Richard seemed to believe that in order to keep me, he needed to rule me. Early in our relationship, we argued and he called me degrading names. I angrily expressed regret for becoming involved with him, and said, "You will never touch me again. Now, get out." Richard sneered, "I can fuck you whenever I want to." I raised my voice, reiterating that he should leave. Richard pushed me to the floor and sat on me, delivering repeated hard slaps across my face, and then raped me, taunting me with the fact that he could and would do what he liked, when he liked. I actually did feel like conquered property: worthless. The rape ended – at least for the time being – further talk of leaving.

## *Jealousy*

Richard believed that as soon as I was out of his sight, I would find another partner. I was going out nightclubbing with friends one evening, and Richard – who disliked me going out without him for the above reason – insisted that I be home by 10 o'clock. I agreed so that he would permit me to go at all. But I was having a good time, and the alcohol I'd consumed provided hubris about defying him, as well as numbing the fear of the consequences.

At 3 am, I crept into the dark flat, hoping that Richard was asleep. But he was waiting for me; he leapt out of bed, saying, quietly but very angrily, "You bitch. Oh, you fucking bitch. Three o'clock?" He began hitting me, demanding to know whom I'd been with, how many times they'd "fucked" me and whether I'd enjoyed it. Denials were useless. He tore my blouse off, shoved me over to our bed and raped me, asking me if it was as good as what I had ostensibly received from another man that night. He blamed me for being home late; unfortunately I believed him.

This experience is representative of others. Oftentimes, Richard's jealousy was ignited not by an actual situation plus his overactive imagination, but by his need to invent a reason to use violence.

## *Reclaiming ownership*

Ending abusive relationships is documented in research as a risk factor for IPSV (DeKeseredy, 2014). One night, I told Richard to leave, and started packing his things. He punched and slapped me all the way to the bed, telling me that I would never get rid of him. After he raped me, he told me that he would do it again every half hour until he couldn't get an erection anymore – or until I changed my mind about throwing him out. The choice, he said, was mine. I sat crying. After the next half hour was up, he prepared to make good on his threat. I broke; Richard stayed.

After a year with Richard, I split with him, and felt resolute about staying free. For some time, I had stopped believing his promises of change, and had been thinking about how to leave. The final precipitator came when Richard had friends around, and I viewed him making obscene gestures behind me while grinning at his friends. The disrespect and degradation reached critical mass, and I told him it was over. Unsurprisingly, he beat and raped me that night. With each stage of the rape – pulling my underwear off, unzipping himself, and penetrating me – Richard offered me the chance to change my mind. The rape was well under way as I continued to stand my ground, and he suddenly collapsed on top of me, and burst into tears. Rape as a weapon had failed him this time, and Richard would never again use it to force reconciliation. Instead, he brought out other potent weapons like suicide threats, and inducing guilt in me. And, a major problem was that I did feel responsible for his feelings. Despite everything he had done to me, I felt like a cruel person for hurting *him*, but still I would not back down from my decision to end the relationship.

Three weeks later, Richard asked if he could come over and talk. He swore that he did not want to browbeat me. I would admit that by this time, I felt a false sense of confidence – I had never stayed free for that long, and I believed that I could control the situation. After all, wouldn't Richard, being truly scared this time, be on his best behavior? At that point, I had not yet read domestic violence literature that reveals the opposite. So, I agreed. Trapping me in my room, Richard berated and beat me for about six hours, before finally raping me, resulting in the conception of my next child. While I have never regretted electing to continue the pregnancy, it was to give Richard leverage that placed me in his power for longer. It had seemed that the rape was partly punishment for leaving, and partly a bid to prove that even if he could not force me to come back, there was one way in which he could still have power over me. However, I also have reason to believe that Richard intended to impregnate me in order to force reconciliation, perhaps thinking that an impending child might achieve what rape by itself could not. IPSV perpetrators who rape to force pregnancy have been identified (Williamson, 2014); further, when pregnancy results from rape, current and past partners are most frequently the perpetrators (Holmes et al., 1996).

### Power and control issues

Myths about rape tell us that it happens because men are *out of control*. For many perpetrators, Richard included, it is actually a way of *asserting* control (see Chapter 4 for further examples).

Except for the time before I began having sex with Richard, I do not recall a single time when he permitted me to say no to sex. Illness, fatigue, or mood were immaterial. He did sometimes ask, but invariably when I said no, he badgered me for a while, after which he would roll me onto my back and force sex anyway. Unless I resisted, these episodes generally did not entail additional physical violence. If I did resist, he dashed my knuckles against the bedhead, and on one occasion, knocked his forehead into mine. The pain – and fear of making it worse – stunned me into inactivity. On one occasion I did resist him to the point of hurting him. He did not complete the rape, but he beat me so badly I honestly thought he was going to kill me.

If I did not resist physically but otherwise displayed distress, Richard scoffed, saying that I wanted it or else I would have tried harder to stop him. But, as indicated above, we both knew the consequences of further resistance.

Like many batterers (Bancroft, 2003), Richard demanded sex after beating me. This is how a batterer may convince himself that if he can have sex with his partner, he need suffer no consequences of beating her (Russell, 1990). I felt angry at being forced to "make up" in this way, but if I refused, I would still be raped, just more violently. And, acquiescence to sex under these circumstances is not "sex," it is *rape*. It is not consensual when a woman knows she will be beaten for refusal. Further, the perpetrator knows that she knows this. Richard warned, "Don't make me come and get you." Resistance meant being dragged into bed by my hair. Sometimes, while getting on top of me, he made a show of kissing me and saying he was sorry. However, Richard may not have been completely convinced that forcing me into sex neutralized physical violence – afterwards, he always wound his arm around my neck from behind so that I could not leave or move away from him; if I moved even slightly, the arm tightened. This felt like a continuation of the violation, but I was not in a position to insist upon being allowed to get up and shower, smoke a cigarette or do something that might have brought some relief.

The use of rape cemented a sense of power and control for Richard not only physically, but also at psychological levels. In hindsight, I believe he knew that he had captured a bright, attractive, compassionate young woman – a *rara avis* whose wings he would set about systematically breaking so that she would not fly away. Rape was a most efficient tool for Richard to construct a mirror into which I would look and see myself as dirty, ugly, and not worth any better.

### Asserting manhood

Richard would become violent if he felt his manhood had been challenged in any way. I went away with him once, to meet some friends from his past. All were of a violent bent with criminal histories, and after I stood up for myself verbally during an argument, they ridiculed Richard for his apparent inability to control "his" woman. One evening, he disappeared for a few hours. When he came home with a friend, I pretended to be asleep while they talked. The friend lay down on another bed, and Richard got into bed with me. Almost immediately, he attempted to mount me for sex. I was horrified and embarrassed that there was another man in the room. I fought, but to no avail; Richard raped me. The friend was awake, and aware of what was happening. Richard had proven that he could control me. (See Chapter 12 for a discussion of the role of male peer support in IPSV).

## Other assaults

### Other types of sexual violence

Men who rape their partners may also inflict a host of other sexual assaults (Easteal and McOrmond-Plummer, 2006). Richard forced touching and kissing on me, or, to illustrate a point, he would grab my hand and force me to touch his penis. It was a fairly constant culture. He often forced me to stand still while he touched me wherever he pleased; if I flinched, he slapped me. Or he made me strip, once while menacing me with a shard of broken glass.

There were boundary violations – for example, Richard never allowed me privacy to shower, which was something I prized. Suggesting that he remove himself and give me space was dangerous. He physically attacked me in the shower recess for doing so.

Bancroft (2003) writes about abusers who use crass, demeaning language that can feel like a sexual assault to their partners. Richard once said, "If you embarrass me in front of my friends, I'll hold you down and let them fuck you. *I* won't even fuck you first." Another example: I had a job at a Chinese restaurant; I came home to Richard asking if I liked sucking "yellow dick." After the end of the relationship, I reflected that it was nice not being called a "slut" all the time, as Richard had used this and other sexually degrading names on almost a daily basis.

Perpetrators of IPSV may deliberately induce shame in their partners (Wall, 2012). One effective way for Richard to do this to me was with the language he used in the course of rape. Being forced to repeat that I was a "whore who liked his cock" was incredibly humiliating. Sometimes, he uttered words and sounds that indicated his own enjoyment of what he was doing, in a way intended to torment me further. My partner intended rape as an "ultimate insult" (McOrmond-Plummer, 2014, p. 46); words were crucial to that purpose.

## Personal history and beliefs of the abuser

While a discussion of factors that may have contributed to their violence is undoubtedly an important part of understanding perpetrators, please note that it is not intended to be an exercise in excusing them.

### *A childhood grounded in misogyny: Richard's father*

It bears stating that many men raised with domestic violence do not abuse their partners. Ineluctably, however, men raised by fathers who disrespect their mothers *may* accept that this defines manhood, and how one relates to women (Bancroft, 2003).

We'll call Richard's mother and father, respectively, Brenda and Jeff. Jeff was an alcoholic with a 20-year history of beating Brenda, whom I remember as terrified of him. Richard told me many disturbing stories (corroborated by his elder sister). What really stood out about Jeff was the way he spoke about women; denigrating them was his default position. I witnessed Jeff calling Brenda a "fucking slut" because she had not put his beer glass out for him to come home to. I heard him tell his 8-year-old daughter that she would be a "slut just like her mother." He frequently informed Richard that I had been "had by everybody." To Jeff, women were concupiscent creatures who, if not sufficiently controlled, would be trading sexual favors with other men. In Richard's presence, he threatened to cut Brenda "from her cunt up to her tits" if he caught her with anybody else. Perhaps it is a fair – and educated – guess that Jeff raped Brenda, and that Richard either witnessed or heard it.

Richard's relationship with his mother was one of love, frustrated protective-ness, withering contempt, and rage. Brenda had been unable to stand up to Jeff when he abused Richard. As he was beating me one night, I held my hands up and pleaded with him not to hurt me anymore. Richard snarled, "Look at you, cowering and cringing just like my fucking stupid bitch mother."

The way Jeff related to Richard was revealing. From Richard's early boy-hood, Jeff had called him a "poofter" (derogatory British and Australian term for a male homosexual) in response to any displays of emotion or sensitivity. I heard him referring to Richard with terms like "girl." Anything remotely associated with the feminine – such as empathy and emotional honesty – was treated with utmost derision. Richard's relationship with Jeff seemed to be a mixture of hating him, fearing him, and yet trying to impress him.

The assimilation of Jeff's views about women was terrifyingly clear in Richard's violence. Most of the rape and sexual assault he perpetrated against me felt like the expression of contempt for me as a *woman* (which is, of course, inherent in gendered crime). To clarify my meaning: I was not anally raped, or even threatened with it. While this is a common form of IPSV used for maximum humiliation of a woman (Finkelhor and Yllo, 1985; Russell, 1990), I believe Richard was more interested in debasing the specifically *female* parts of my body – breasts and vagina. I remember him saying "I'm going to hurt you inside so you will never want another man." The rapes did feel sometimes as if he was trying to injure me physically as well as psychologically, like a metaphorical stabbing at my womanhood.

Richard did have a sad childhood in which he learned appalling and extremely dangerous lessons about women and about what being a man is. However, he also knew, and often expressed, that what Jeff had done to Brenda was wrong. Unfortunately, this did not translate into Richard changing his own behavior. Bancroft (2003) writes that although many abusive men promise change, they do not ultimately wish to relinquish the benefits they accrue through intimidating women. It was evident to me that Richard relished the power that violence gave him.

### Belief in the Madonna/whore dichotomy

Diana Russell writes, "In Western societies there are still 'good girls' and 'bad girls,' virgins and whores. And male behavior toward females generally depends on which of the two labels females are perceived to deserve" (1975, p. 25). Richard espoused a very strong view of women as either Madonnas or whores, but in a relationship, this dichotomy could exist for him in the same woman. When I met him he placed me on a pedestal. This was embarrassing, because I knew perfectly well that I was not the angel he had designated me as. While he perceived me as the "Madonna," his treatment of me was almost slavish. When I tumbled from that lofty but completely unrealistic ideal and became, in his view, the "whore," punishment was swift. Becoming the "whore" might mean I wore something that made it too obvious I had breasts, or that another man had admired me. At these times, Richard told me as he raped me, that he was doing it to teach me not to be a "slut," because this is what sluts get. He would mock me with a syrupy crooning – the memory of which is still faintly nauseating: "Aw, what's the matter, baby? Sluts like it, and you're a slut, aren't you? I'm just giving you what sluts want." We see in Chapter 4 how perpetrators may subscribe to such myths because it helps them justify their abuses; Richard was no exception.

### Eroticizing of sexual violence

I have said above that Richard usually used sexual violence to meet nonsexual needs. Sometimes, though, the rape itself did appear to be sexually arousing for him. When we first became intimate, Richard confessed sexual fantasies about rape. He said he found the idea exciting. He told me that he had once followed a woman with the intention of raping her, and then had thought, "What has that poor bitch ever done to me?" (This is perhaps revealing, as if anything she could have done would have justified raping her. At least Richard seemed to have no confusion that it was a bad thing to do.) At the time, I was glad to hear that he had not done it, and told him that I had been raped at fourteen. He seemed genuinely sympathetic and angry with the perpetrator. I did not know then that this "protective" attitude suggested an ownership that would be ultimately dangerous, or that he would find my vulnerability attractive. In hindsight, it occurred to me that this conversation may have been a form of *grooming*, or assessing my vulnerabilities for later use.

On occasions when Richard raped me, it was as if he was acting out an internal script of what, based on his fantasies (and perhaps a diet of bad B-movies), he thought a rapist should be. Some men do eroticize rape, because for them, the inherent domination over women that rape is, equates with virility and power (Bancroft, 2003; see more in Chapter 4). I am persuaded to believe that if I had not been such a "safe" victim, Richard would have raped other women. He *liked* rape, and the power it accrued him.

## Endings

After two years, I decided I had to break free for good. With separation, Richard was particularly enraged that I might meet somebody else. He beat me and on occasion sexually assaulted me, jamming fingers in my vagina, asking who I was "fucking" and whether their penis was better than his. He often used the pretext of having rights to visit his child, in whom he was not actually interested at all. And I did not dare deny him entry to my home; I knew he would simply kick the door in. At this time, rape was no longer so much an expedient to subjugation as it was simply a means to remind me that he still had the power to do it. The death threats grew worse – Richard's mother warned me that he was likely to kill me. Late one night, he arrived with a knife and menaced me with it for hours, sexually assaulting me periodically, and forcing me to say I loved him. This ended when I instigated sex with him – to save myself. This was not the first time I had bartered my body for (relative) safety. Richard had told me, "I came here tonight to kill you. I was going to kill you." It was (and still is) apparent to me that he had actually resolved to do so that night.

When Richard held my head under a bathtub full of water, saying that he would never share me, I knew I had to act before he really did kill me, though I was by no means certain that any action would help. I applied for custody of my baby, and for a restraining order. Richard responded that unless I dropped the whole thing and reconciled with him, he would have me declared unfit as a mother, and take the child. I have never forgotten his words: "If you mention the rape, I'll make it look like child's play. Call my bluff, bitch." In my love for my children I found the strength to move forward, and got both custody and the restraining order. I was grateful to be alive, and Richard became heavily involved in heroin use, eventually losing all interest in contact.

## The relationship between rape and homicide

The fact that battering perpetrators of IPSV are likely to murder their victims is expanded upon more fully in Chapter 2. I faced many credible homicidal threats and behaviors from Richard; in addition to those detailed above, he strangled me, smothered me with a pillow, and threatened me with a hunting rifle. My fears that he was capable of murder were borne out when, after the relationship concluded, Richard was sentenced and incarcerated for the particularly brutal murder of a drugs associate. What follows is how I view the connection between rape and murder, based on my experiences.

### Entitlement

It seems to me that killing a partner stems from the same root of entitlement as raping a partner. When a violent man rapes his partner, he feels that she is his property to dispense with as he wishes. Richard's homicidal threats and actions had the same feel: If I would not live with him, I would not live at all – and he had the *right* to make that decision.

### Possession and sexual jealousy

Adams's work *Why do they kill?* (2007) provides some grotesque and truly frightening examples of attitudes of sexual ownership in femicidal men: "John," who raped and murdered his estranged wife Debra, reported that the act of rape before murder was a way of letting Debra's new partner know that John had been the "last to have her" (Adams, 2007, p. 209). John felt that sex before killing his ex-partner was "a way of preserving us as a couple forever" (Adams, 2007, p. 50). It will be evident from descriptions I have given above, that sexual jealousy and asserting ownership were common elements underpinning Richard's sexual assaults. His murderous gestures also contained these elements; he had frequently made threats such as "If you ever go out with anybody else, I will kill you." This was often followed by such statements as "You're mine. I will never let you go." Richard's sexual jealousy became especially dangerous once he understood that I was definitely not going to reconcile with him, as illustrated by his declaring that he would never share me before holding my head underwater.

## Objectification

Rape is both contributed to by, and contributes to, denial of a woman's personhood, reducing her to the status of a *thing* – "bitch," "whore," or "cunt." Prior to rape and/or murderous threats, Richard used such language to deliberately objectify me as a *dirty* thing so that he didn't have to feel bad about hurting me. And, as Adams argues in Chapter 2, acts of sexual assault serve to further perpetuate the perpetrator's objectification of his victim; this may be why some men rape their ex/partners before killing them, and is one reason why IPSV is a fatality risk factor. For Richard, murdering me would have been the logical step for somebody who spent time justifying both before sexual abuse and *because* of it, that it was perfectly acceptable to do what one will with a "thing" – somebody who is not actually a person with rights.

## Devaluation

In the case of rape or death threats, Richard could switch very quickly from pleading and cajoling to violence. As he pleaded, and did not get what he wanted, the shifting of his mental gears was perceptible: "You're only a bitch anyway, forcing me to crawl to you. Fuck you." He seemed to perceive a campaign to reconcile as a sort of favor, which, once refused, made violence justifiable.

## Power

As this chapter indicates, Richard used rape as the ultimate way of breaking me when other means failed. If beating me didn't work, rape was the only way left to establish power. When even this ceased to work, threats to my life became the final power that he could have.

## Further considerations

### Did Richard love me?

Aphrodite Matsakis (1994) writes that some abusers do love their partners, or are able to show love to them when they are not being abusive. Richard could be intensely loving, but only for as long as he did not become angry and decide I deserved to be hurt. Perhaps the real question is how an abuser defines love. For Richard, love was ownership, and entrapment of somebody with fear and pity. And, rape is certainly not an act of love.

### Remorse?

For his physical abuse, Richard sometimes did express remorse, which may have been genuine for the moment, but it did not last. He rarely expressed remorse for the rapes; generally, they were not spoken about, and I was definitely anxious to pretend that something which felt so shameful had not happened. The morning after a bad night, Richard would scan me for signs of a response. If I so much as tightened my bath towel because I did not want him to see me naked, it provoked him and he reminded me of why the rape was my fault.

On one occasion, however, Richard had beaten me into submission before a particularly vicious rape. He stopped suddenly and held me, saying that he was sorry, then he gently helped me into the shower. Two other times when he was threatening me with rape, he also stopped, and entreating me to stop crying, said that he hadn't really been going to do it. Perhaps something occasionally stirred within Richard – too little too late – but I am not sure that it constituted actual remorse. True remorse would have been to confront his behavior, and Richard did not want this. Once, I told him that I was struggling with the sexual abuse. He gave me one of the worst beatings I remember, and said, "If you ever mention that again, I'll kill you."

Having my abuser also be my comforter caused further entrapment, and created conditions for traumatic bonding (see Chapter 7).

### Did Richard know it was rape?

In the study of Parkinson and Cowan (2008), no IPSV perpetrator viewed the act as criminal. This is often due to issues like perceived entitlement to a partner's body.

Richard seemed to know (more clearly than I did) that what he was doing was rape, but perhaps saw it as not quite "real" rape since I was his partner. I suggested reporting him once, and he laughed at me, saying, "I've fucked you so many times – who will believe you?" However he viewed it, what seems truly chilling about Richard is how thoroughly he knew that rape was a means of seriously hurting a woman and making her feel reduced. Knowing this, he used rape with a conscious deliberation.

### What was sex like otherwise?

Sex with Richard, when he wasn't being abusive, was quite normal. He could be quite reverential about the same body he abused on other occasions. I believe that this was one way in which he compartmentalized his abusiveness.

   He often used the "normal" sex against me. For example, if one night held consensual sex and the next night held rape, Richard taunted me, saying, "You liked it last night." He was not confused. He knew perfectly well that raping me was not the same as consensual and enjoyed sex. He intended to shame me, and make me feel responsible for the rape.

### Was Richard mentally ill?

Although it is a common belief that somebody who commits rape must be "sick," this is not usually the case (Russell, 1990). In particular, when an abuser turns fatal and murders his partner, the media frequently makes assertions about mental illness. This misses the crucial point that mental illness is not so much a causative factor in partner abuse as the sense of a right to control women (Bancroft, 2003). Richard did not generally appear to suffer from any mental illness except for perhaps some depression when the relationship concluded. While it is known that a depressed perpetrator may be a risk factor for fatality (Campbell et al., 2003), the underlying and far more dangerous "disease" is the entitlement I have referred to above. It is vital that any consideration of mental illness in perpetrators does not become another way to absolve them of responsibility for deliberately chosen and executed crimes.

### What about substance abuse/addictions?

Richard used amphetamines and alcohol during the relationship, but on a periodic basis only – he had not yet progressed to full-blown addiction. It is true that the beatings, which were bad enough when he was sober, tended to worsen when he was drunk. However, I recall very few instances of rape – either the physically violent or the verbally coercive – in which Richard was under the influence of either drugs or alcohol. Bancroft (2003) sounds a warning about the dangers of over-focusing on substance abuse in violent men, cautioning that a perpetrator who may receive treatment for these issues simply becomes a sober perpetrator, with his perception of entitlement to control women still well and truly intact. While substance abuse may sometimes be a contributing factor, it is, again, not an excuse.

## Conclusion

When one has been where I have, being alive feels most fortunate – especially when we consider how many women who have shared similar journeys to me have been murdered. I have thus been pleased to have an opportunity to set out a bird's-eye view of what somebody who beats, rapes, and has terrifyingly real potential to kill his partner may look like.

Women being raped and beaten must be made aware of the risk to their lives. Awareness is crucial, and as such it is my hope that this chapter helps facilitate recognition of the Richards of the world, and the formulation of appropriate interventions. We must also hold them accountable, because the horrifyingly common occurrence of IPSV (Myhill & Allen, 2002) indicates that men are committing such crimes against partners frequently and with impunity. Just as importantly, I want this chapter to aid understanding, response, and improvements in legal protection for women living with men like Richard – before they are dead.

## References

Adams, D. (2007). *Why do they kill? Men who murder their intimate partners*. Nashville, TN: Vanderbilt University Press.

Bancroft, L. (2003). *Why does he do that? Inside the minds of angry and controlling men*. New York, NY: Berkeley Publishing Group.

Campbell, J.C., Webster, D., Koziol-McLain, J., Block, C.R., Campbell, D., Curry, M., Gary, F., McFarlane, J., Sachs, C., Sharps, P., Ulrich, Y., & Wilt, S.A. (2003). Assessing risk factors for intimate partner homicide. *National Institutes of Justice Journal*, 250, 14–19.

DeKeseredy, W. (2014). Separation/divorce sexual assault. In L. McOrmond Plummer, P. Easteal, & J.Y. Levy-Peck, *Intimate partner sexual violence* (pp. 65–75). London, UK: Jessica Kingsley Publishers.

Easteal, P., & McOrmond-Plummer, L. (2006). *Real rape, real pain*. Melbourne, Australia: Hybrid Press.

Finkelhor, D., & Yllo, K. (1985). *License to rape: Sexual abuse of wives*. New York, NY: The Free Press.

Holmes, M.M., Resick, H.S., Kilpatrick, D.G., & Best, C.L. (1996). Rape-related pregnancy: Estimates and descriptive characteristics from a national sample of women. *American Journal of Obstetrics and Gynecology*, *175*(2), 320–325.

McOrmond-Plummer, L. (2014). Considering the differences: Intimate partner sexual violence in sexual assault and domestic violence discourse. In L. McOrmond-Plummer, P. Easteal, & J.Y. Levy-Peck (Eds.), *Intimate partner sexual violence: A multidisciplinary guide to improving services and support for survivors of rape and abuse* (pp. 41–53). London, UK: Jessica Kingsley Publishers.

Matsakis, A. (1992). *I can't get over it: A handbook for trauma survivors*. Oakland, CA: New Harbinger Publications.

Myhill, A. & Allen, J. (2002) *Rape and sexual assault of women: Findings from the British crime survey*. London, UK: Home Office. Retrieved from: www.aphroditewounded.org/Myhill and Allen.pdf.

Parkinson, D., & Cowan, S. (2008). *Raped by a partner: Nowhere to go, no-one to tell.* Victoria, Australia: Women's Health Goulburn North East.

Russell, D. (1975). *The politics of rape: The victim's perspective.* New York, NY: Stein and Day.

Russell, D. (1990). *Rape in marriage.* New York, NY: Macmillan Publishing Company.

Wall, L. (2012, January). *The many facets of shame in intimate partner sexual violence. ACSSA Research Summary.* Melbourne, Australia: Australian Centre for the Study of Sexual Assault.

Williamson, E. (2014). Reproductive coercion. In L. McOrmond-Plummer, P. Easteal, & J.Y. Levy-Peck (Eds.), *Intimate partner sexual violence: A multidisciplinary guide to improving services and support for survivors of rape and abuse* (pp. 76–85). London, UK: Jessica Kingsley Publishers.

Wilson, K.J. (1997). *When violence begins at home: A comprehensive guide to understanding and ending domestic violence.* Alameda, CA: Hunter House Publishers.

# Chapter 11

# Perpetrators and reproductive coercion

*Jennifer Y. Levy-Peck*

## Overview

When two individuals become a couple, they often make decisions about reproductive issues, such as whether to have a child. Even in a loving, egalitarian relationship, these decisions can be difficult, because the stakes are high and it is hard to compromise: you either have a child, or you don't, for example. In a relationship based on coercive control by one partner over the other (as is typical in cases of intimate partner sexual violence), these decisions are often not mutual. In fact, decisions about reproductive issues may be particularly likely to be subject to power tactics. Evan Stark (2009), who coined the term "coercive control," explains that "many of the regulations involved in coercive control target behaviors that are identified with the female role" (p. 15). Certainly, pregnancy, childbirth, breastfeeding, and child-rearing are intimately identified with the female role in our society, and thus may become the focus of abusive, controlling behavior.

## What is reproductive coercion?

The American College of Obstetricians and Gynecologists (2013, p. 1) provides this definition:

> Reproductive and sexual coercion involves behavior intended to maintain power and control in a relationship related to reproductive health by someone who is, was, or wishes to be involved in an intimate or dating relationship with an adult or adolescent. This behavior includes explicit attempts to impregnate a partner against her will, control outcomes of a pregnancy, coerce a partner to have unprotected sex, and interfere with contraceptive methods.

## Forms of reproductive coercion

These terms come from the work of a group of researchers affiliated with Futures Without Violence (Chamberlain & Levenson, 2011).

**Birth control sabotage**, a common form of reproductive coercion, consists of interfering with birth control. For example, an abusive partner may throw out contraceptive pills, poke holes in condoms, or even forcibly remove a partner's intrauterine device (IUD).

**Pregnancy pressure** occurs when a partner uses physical or verbal abuse or coercion to insist that his reluctant partner become pregnant. For example, he may tell her that he will leave her or have a baby with another woman if she does not become pregnant, or he may actually rape her in order to force a pregnancy.

**Pregnancy coercion** involves forcing an unwanted outcome once a woman does become pregnant – for example, threatening a partner with physical harm if she does not have an abortion, forcing a woman to carry a pregnancy to term, or beating her to the point where she has a miscarriage.

**Sexual coercion related to reproductive health** may involve a man refusing to use a condom or deliberately trying to infect his partner with a sexually transmitted infection (STI) or HIV. Some men retaliate violently when informed that their partner has an STI (even if they may have infected her) (Decker et al., 2011). Others insist that their partners must not use contraception, going so far as to keep track of the women's menstrual cycles or manually checking for the presence of an IUD (Chamberlain & Levenson, 2011).

## Relationship between reproductive health and intimate partner violence

Box 11.1 summarizes strategies of reproductive coercion along with abusive behaviors that focus on reproductive health issues.

### Abortion

Silverman and colleagues (2010) undertook a study of more than 1,300 young men ages 18–35 recruited from community health centers in urban, low-income areas. Nearly one-third of the participants had perpetrated physical or sexual violence against a female partner, by their own accounts. Of those men who reported having perpetrated violence, almost half (48.9%) said that they had been involved in a pregnancy that ended in abortion, compared to 26% of those who did not report having been violent. The men who reported perpetrating violence were also more likely to have been involved in three or more abortions. Nearly 20% of the men who had been abusive reported that there had been conflict with their partners about whether or not to have an abortion, compared to 7% of the nonabusive men. These conflicts involved both types of outcomes – that is, some men wanted their reluctant partners to

## Box 11.1  Reproductive coercion and intimate partner violence

### REPRODUCTIVE HEALTH

**BIRTH CONTROL SABOTAGE**

- Accusing a woman of infidelity if she wants to use birth control
- Telling a woman that birth control will ruin her future fertility
- Hiding, throwing away, or destroying birth control
- Pulling out contraceptive rings
- Pulling off contraceptive patches
- Poking holes in condoms
- Refusing to pull out during sex when previously agreed upon
- Refusing to use condoms
- Breaking/removing condoms during sex
- Physically or economically preventing a woman from obtaining birth control

**PREGNANCY PRESSURE**

- Pressuring a woman to get pregnant when she does not want to
- Threatening to hurt a woman physically, economically, or emotionally if she refuses to get pregnant
- Making a woman feel guilty for not wanting to become pregnant
- Accusing a woman of infidelity if she refuses to get pregnant
- Claiming that a woman must not be "in love" if she does not want to become pregnant

**PREGNANCY OUTCOME CONTROL**

- Forcing/pressuring a woman to continue a pregnancy or have an abortion against her will
- Making a woman feel guilty for wanting to continue a pregnancy or have an abortion
- Hurting a woman (or threatening to hurt a woman) physically and/or emotionally if she continues a pregnancy or has an abortion
- Physically assaulting a woman in an attempt to induce a miscarriage

### INTIMATE PARTNER VIOLENCE

**PHYSICAL ABUSE [note: also sexual]**

- Beating, kicking, hitting, strangling, or using any form of physical violence to force a woman to become pregnant, continue a pregnancy, or have an abortion
- Purposefully harming a woman so that she miscarries, delivers early, or ends up having a child requiring special assistance
- Hurting or threatening to hurt others to force a woman to choose a particular pregnancy outcome
- Destroying a woman's property or possessions to pressure her to comply with his reproductive wishes
- Raping a woman to get her pregnant

**ECONOMIC ABUSE**

- Refusing to help pay for birth control or an abortion
- Refusing to help with the costs of raising the child (or other shared children) if a woman continues a pregnancy
- Refusing to help pay for prenatal care and basic health needs if a woman continues a pregnancy
- Forcing pregnancies and births, one after another within a short time frame, so that she is unable to work or leave the home without difficulty or risk
- Destroying a woman's credit, sabotaging assets, or amassing debt in an attempt to force her to have a baby, or get an abortion
- Sabotaging a woman's ability to earn her own income in an attempt to force her to have a baby, or get an abortion

**EMOTIONAL ABUSE**

- Convincing a woman that no other person would want her if she chooses a certain pregnancy outcome
- Calling a woman names, degrading her, or using profanity directed at her, in an effort to coerce her to choosing a certain pregnancy outcome
- Threatening to harm oneself, or others, to coerce a woman into choose a certain pregnancy outcome
- Threatening to hurt/kill a woman if she does not choose a certain pregnancy outcome
- Threatening to "out" a woman for an incident/choice/behavior she may want to remain secret if she does not choose a certain pregnancy outcome
- Using a woman's religious or cultural beliefs to manipulate her into choosing a certain pregnancy outcome

Source: From *Exposing Reproductive Coercion Toolkit*, available at: www.ncdv.org/files/RCtoolkit.pdf. Used by kind permission of the National Coalition Against Domestic Violence.

obtain an abortion, while others wanted their partners to continue the pregnancy. The researchers state:

> Although these cross-sectional analyses did not allow us to reach definitive conclusions regarding causal relationships, the findings from previous research suggest that these results likely reflected abusive men's greater involvement in unintended pregnancy, stemming from a range of behaviors that include forced or coerced sex, condom refusal, and control over contraception . . . These data describe the significant threat to women's reproductive control related to violence from male partners, a threat that should be considered in the design of all services and policies related to family planning and abortion.
>
> (Silverman et al., 2010, p. 1416)

### Forced pregnancy as a control measure

Much of the information available about perpetrators of forced pregnancy is in the form of documents and research reports regarding forced pregnancy being used as a form of genocide in ethnic conflicts worldwide. In fact, historians and political scientists note that " 'forced impregnation' has been used throughout history as a tool of assimilation or subjugation of the enemy, minority, or slave populations" (Carpenter, 2000, p. 233). In the global context, it becomes clear that sexual violence and pregnancy coercion intersect as methods of abuse and control: "If a woman is raped and forced to carry the child of the rapist, then the creation of that child involved violations of her human rights" (Carpenter, 2000, p. 222).

Yet there is surprisingly little attention to pregnancy as a consequence of partner rape. In McFarlane and colleagues' study of IPSV (2005), 20% of the women reported a rape-related pregnancy. Of women who became pregnant (with or without rape), 31% were also subjected to sexual violence during pregnancy. Only 16% of the rape-related pregnancies ended in abortion; it is unknown whether or not this was influenced by pregnancy coercion by the partner.

If a survivor of IPSV decides to separate from her partner after a rape resulting in conception, she may enter a minefield of legal issues involving the child, including custody and visitation battles that prolong the perpetrator's control over her life and that of the child (Bitar, 2012). In the U.S., there is a patchwork quilt of legislation that does little to create a clear boundary between a rapist father and his victim. Silver (2014) describes this lack of legal protection as a "second rape":

> the legal system and state legislatures have bound the rape victim through the child to the rapist, thereby becoming complicit in what can be viewed as a "second rape." This secondary victimization occurs when the rapist

manipulates the omission of legal protections and asserts parental rights in order to control and traumatize his victim for a second time. (section VII)

Emotionally and financially, the survivor may feel more tightly bound to the perpetrator after an unintended pregnancy, and this may be the perpetrator's intent (Easteal & McOrmond-Plummer, 2006).

Rapid repeat pregnancy, which is defined as pregnancy within 12 to 24 months of a previous pregnancy, is associated with intimate partner violence and is particularly problematic for adolescent mothers (Raneri & Wiemann, 2007), who suffer educational and economic consequences that make it more difficult for them to move forward in life.

### Forced noncondom use

Purdie, Abbey, and Jaques-Tiura (2010) studied men who forced female partners to have sex without a condom. The authors cite previous work by Raj and colleagues (Raj et al., 2006; Santana, Raj, Decker, La Marche, & Silverman, 2006) who studied 283 sexually active male patients (18–35 years old) at an urban community health center. These men all had steady dating partners, and nearly a quarter (24%) of the men stated that they had forced a partner to have sex without a condom. Purdie and colleagues' 2010 study included 78 college men who indicated that they had used coercive methods to force a dating partner to have sex. Approximately half of these individuals did not use a condom. The researchers compared this group with the men who did use condoms, and concluded:

> Perpetrators who made a dating partner have unprotected sex were more accepting of using verbal pressure against women, held more positive attitudes toward casual sex, had sexual intercourse more frequently, had physically assaulted a dating partner more frequently (marginal effect), and more frequently injured their dating partner than perpetrators who had not made a dating partner have unprotected sex. There were no differences in sexual dominance or alcohol consumption during sexual situations.
>
> (p. 1091)

Thus the study results bore out the hypothesis that perpetrators who forced sex without a condom exhibited a greater desire to control their female partners. The authors considered the results as preliminary, but as highlighting the need to consider sexual violence when looking to prevent the risk of STI transmission and unintended pregnancy. The researchers also make the important point that women who have been in sexually coercive or violent relationships may not feel comfortable negotiating condom use, even with a subsequent nonaggressive partner, and thus men who respect their partners' wishes may need to take extra care in discussing this issue with survivors of previous IPSV.

## Interference with Breastfeeding

Considerably more research is needed to determine definitively whether IPSV has a negative effect on a new mother's ability to breastfeed. While studies have shown that women who experience any form of intimate partner violence during pregnancy or after childbirth are less likely to breastfeed their babies, it appears that other factors (such as being single, black, or a smoker) have more predictive power than the presence of IPV alone (Silverman, Decker, Reed, & Raj, 2006).

However, there is a need for qualitative and quantitative research looking at whether IPSV perpetration interferes with a woman's willingness or ability to breastfeed. Certainly, IPSV perpetrators' desire for power and control over a woman's sexual self might reasonably be assumed to create a hostile atmosphere when a new mother wants to use her breasts for something other than her partner's sexual satisfaction. The emotional abuse and body shaming that IPSV perpetrators place upon their partners may also make it difficult for survivors to muster the self-confidence to breastfeed.

One of the few studies to look specifically at sexual IPV and breastfeeding is Misch and Yount's (2014) study of women in eight African nations. They state:

> . . . we discovered that the most common association across countries was that between sexual IPV victimization and suboptimal breastfeeding, especially less exclusive breastfeeding in Ghana, Kenya, and Liberia. . . . because breastfeeding involves the function of a sometimes sexualized organ, sexual IPV victimization may result in an acute aversion to early and exclusive breastfeeding. Given that sexual IPV victimization was associated with suboptimal breastfeeding more often than the other forms of IPV victimization, experiencing sexual objectification and victimization may be a more powerful pathway of effect than those associated with emotional and physical IPV.
>
> (p. 696)

# Strategies to address perpetrators of reproductive coercion

## Focus on primary prevention

Loving, violence-free relationships are a benefit to all, and the best way to address perpetration is to try to prevent it in the first place. Comprehensive sex education should include information about consent, boundaries, shared responsibility for contraception and sexually transmitted infection prevention, and the impact of unintended pregnancy on both parents' lives. Reproductive coercion can only truly be prevented by an overall approach to enhance gender equity, nonviolent and noncoercive conflict resolution, and respect within relationships (see Chapter 20 for more information on prevention issues).

### Protect health care settings

Perpetrators should not be allowed to intimidate survivors who are seeking health care, particularly reproductive health care. For example, in a healthy, respectful relationship it may be desirable for the father to accompany a pregnant woman during her obstetrician appointments; but if the father is abusive, his presence may prevent the woman from receiving appropriate care and help. This is also true in an abortion clinic or at contraceptive appointments. A reasonable way to handle this concern is to see the patient alone in the examining room for a portion of each appointment, even if her partner accompanies her. This can be done as part of the routine, and explained as "policy." Futures Without Violence offers training videos on their website (www.futureswithoutviolence.org) to help medical clinicians see how to do this in a comfortable and respectful manner. This practice can also help clinicians to offer birth control that is less detectable by a controlling partner, without the partner's knowledge.

Health care providers should consider the possibility that a perpetrator may compromise a patient's safety during any interaction. For example, information about advocacy services should be provided in private areas (rest rooms and examining rooms) and in small formats (such as business-card-size materials) so that perpetrators are less likely to discover and retaliate when patients view or take these materials. Another safety strategy is to offer victim advocacy services within medical clinics, so perpetrators may not find out that their partners are receiving these services.

### Create opportunities for conversation

In addition to primary prevention, professionals should offer opportunities to discuss inappropriate and abusive behavior, and outline the consequences of that behavior. In general, professionals are becoming more skilled in identifying and interacting with survivors, but we still often fail to address those who perpetrate coercive behaviors or are at risk of doing so.

Parents and peers (of any age) certainly have an important role in these conversations as well. A parent may consider, "Would my son know what to say to a friend who thinks that getting a girl pregnant is a sign of manhood?" "Does my son think this way himself, and if so, what information does he need to understand this is not true?"

Teachers, health care providers, coaches, and extended family members should also be alert to conversational openings to discuss a supportive and respectful approach to the reproductive needs and choices of one's partner. College students and other adults can confront controlling behaviors and attitudes by their friends.

## Break stereotypes of abusers

Reproductive coercion can be employed by anyone, and it usually occurs in private settings. As with other forms of IPSV, professionals who think they "know" what an abuser looks like or acts like in a public setting are deluding themselves. Professionals who work with survivors of any form of physical, emotional, or sexual abuse, or who provide any reproductive health care, should consider that reproductive coercion may be part of the picture.

## Lessen abusers' power

While many friends, family members, and professionals pressure survivors to leave abusive and coercive partners, this strategy may backfire. While offering support and protective strategies to those who do want to leave the relationship is critical, it is also vital to recognize that many survivors are going to remain in ongoing abusive relationships, at least for some period of time, and those survivors also need strategies to enhance their safety and options for the future. Because unintended pregnancy and childbearing has such a huge impact on a woman's life – including her employment, housing, and financial opportunities – and can bind her more firmly to an abusive partner, strategies such as having emergency contraception on hand, offering access to abortion services, and providing less detectable birth control can undermine the abuser's power while his partner remains in the relationship (Washington State Attorney General, Washington Coalition of Sexual Assault Programs, & Washington State Coalition Against Domestic Violence, 2013). Laws and policies that limit women's access to these services or require approval by her partner can perpetuate abusive situations.

Most reproductive coercion will fall under the radar of the criminal justice system. It is not a crime to tell your girlfriend that you will find someone else if she won't have your baby. It is not a crime to insist on an abortion. Those behaviors that *do* rise to the level of a criminal offense, such as yanking out an intrauterine contraceptive device or physically restraining a partner from going to an advocacy meeting, are unlikely to be reported and pursued for criminal remedies. The tools at our disposal are robust prevention programs, protection of survivors in service settings, education of the public and of professionals, and advocacy services that specifically address reproductive coercion.

## Consider the role of IPSV and reproductive coercion in unplanned pregnancy

Adolescent mothers are often studied, discussed, and provided services as though they became pregnant on their own. Similarly, the broader issue of unintended pregnancy is frequently considered only in terms of contraceptive knowledge and access. Programs and policies to address teen and unplanned pregnancy must also address IPSV and reproductive coercion, and focus on ways to reduce perpetration.

### Include reproductive coercion issues in batterers' treatment

Those who commit reproductive coercion are not necessarily all considered "batterers," in the sense of having perpetrated physical violence, but certainly a proportion of physical abusers also use sexual and reproductive coercion as methods of control. More research is needed on effective interventions to eliminate these strategies along with other forms of abuse in intimate partner relationships. Batterer treatment programs should include these topics and find ways to reduce behaviors related to reproductive coercion.

## Directions for further research

As with other aspects of IPSV, most research in the field of reproductive coercion focuses on the victim rather than the perpetrator. Elizabeth Miller and her colleagues, some of the preeminent researchers on reproductive coercion, identify some of the many questions that remain to be answered:

> . . . does partner violence manifest before attempts to control a woman's pregnancy and the outcomes of that pregnancy? Or do coercive behaviors that include attempts to control her body and reproductive outcomes foreshadow physical and sexual violence in the relationship? And related to this, why might men engage in such controlling behaviors? How do they recognize and understand reproductive coercion? And finally, what might we do to reduce the prevalence of this range of behaviors among young men?
>
> (Miller, Jordan, Levenson, & Silverman, 2010, p. 458)

While the study cited above focused on young men, I would add that research about reduction of reproductive coercion should focus on *all* those who engage in this behavior.

## Conclusion

Reproductive coercion is a tool for limiting a partner's freedom. It may occur in conjunction with other forms of IPSV, such as partner rape, or separately, but in any case it restricts women's choices and has a negative impact on their health. We need to turn the lens of scrutiny on perpetrators and those at risk for perpetration to address this global concern.

# References

American College of Obstetricians and Gynecologists, Committee on Health Care for Underserved Women. (2013). Reproductive and sexual coercion. *Committee Opinion*, Number 225 (February). Retrieved from: www.acog.org/Resources-And-Publications/Committee-Opinions/Committee-on-Health-Care-for-Underserved-Women/Reproductive-and-Sexual-Coercion.

Bitar, K.N. (2012). The parental rights of rapists. *Duke Journal of Gender Law & Policy, 19*, 275.

Carpenter, R.C. (2000). Forced maternity, children's rights and the genocide convention: A theoretical analysis. *Journal of Genocide Research, 2*(2), 213–244. doi: 10.1080/713677603.

Chamberlain, L., & Levenson, R. (2011). *Reproductive health and partner violence guidelines: An integrated response to intimate partner violence and reproductive and sexual coercion* (2nd ed.). San Francisco, CA: Futures Without Violence.

Decker, M.R., Miller, E., McCauley, H.L., Tancredi, D.J., Levenson, R.R., Waldman J., Schoenwald, P., Silverman J.G. (2011). Intimate partner violence and partner notification of sexually transmitted infections among adolescent and young adult family planning clinic patients. *International Journal of STD & AIDS, 22*(6), 345–347. doi:10.1258/ijsa.2011.010425.

Easteal, P., & McOrmond-Plummer, L. (2006). *Real rape, real pain: Help for women sexually assaulted by male partners.* Melbourne, Australia: Hybrid Press.

McFarlane, J., Malecha, A., Watson, K., Gist, J., Batten, E., Hall, I., & Smith, S. (2005). Intimate partner sexual assault against women: Frequency, health consequences, and treatment outcomes. *Journal of Obstetrics and Gynecology, 105*, 99–108.

Miller, E., Jordan, B., Levenson, R., & Silverman, J.G. (2010). Reproductive coercion: Connecting the dots between partner violence and unintended pregnancy. *Contraception, 81*(6), 457–459. doi.org/10.1016/j.contraception.2010.02.023.

Misch, E.S., & Yount, K.M. (2014). Intimate partner violence and breastfeeding in Africa. *Maternal and Child Health Journal, 18*(3), 688–697. doi:10.1007/s10995-013-1294-x.

Purdie, M.P., Abbey, A., & Jacques-Tiura, A.J. (2010). Perpetrators of intimate partner sexual violence: Are there unique characteristics associated with making partners have sex without a condom? *Violence Against Women, 16*, 1086. doi: 10.1177/107780121038 2859.

Raj, A., Santana, C., La Marche, A., Amaro, H., Cranston, K., & Silverman, J.G. (2006). Perpetration of intimate partner violence associated with sexual risk behaviors among young adult men. *American Journal of Public Health, 96*, 1873–1878.

Raneri, L.G., & Wiemann, C.M. (2007). Social ecological predictors of repeat adolescent pregnancy. *Perspectives on Sexual and Reproductive Health, 39*(1), 39–47.

Santana, M.C., Raj, A., Decker, M.R., La Marche, A., & Silverman, J.G. (2006). Masculine gender roles associated with increased sexual risk and intimate partner violence perpetration among young adult men. *Journal of Urban Health: Bulletin of the New York Academy of Medicine, 83*, 575–585.

Silver, M. (2014). The second rape: Legal options for rape survivors to terminate parental rights. *Family Law Quarterly, 48*(3), 515–537.

Silverman, J.G., Decker, M.R., Reed, E., & Raj, A. (2006). Intimate partner violence around the time of pregnancy: Association with breastfeeding behavior. *Journal of Women's Health, 15*(8), 934–940.

Silverman, J.G., Decker, M.E., McCauley, H.L., Gupta, J., Miller, E., Raj, A., & Goldberg, A.B. (2010). Male perpetration of intimate partner violence and involvement in abortions and abortion-related conflict. *American Journal of Public Health, 100*(8), 1415–1417.

Stark, E. (2009). *Coercive control: How men entrap women in personal life.* New York, NY: Oxford University Press.

Washington State Attorney General, Washington Coalition of Sexual Assault Programs, & Washington State Coalition Against Domestic Violence (2013). An integrated approach to intimate partner violence and reproductive & sexual coercion. Retrieved from: www.pregnantsurvivors.org.

# Part 4

# How perpetrators are condoned

The social context of intimate partner sexual violence

# The role of male peer support in intimate partner sexual violence perpetrators' offending

*Walter S. DeKeseredy*

## Introduction

Intimate partner sexual violence (IPSV), like other forms of woman abuse (e.g., coercive control and battering), can only be curbed through the creation and implementation of policies that target the broader social and social psychological forces that perpetuate and legitimate intimate violence (True, 2012). What are these forces? Of course, it is impossible to simply pick out one "reason" and announce that it covers all cases at all times. Yet, it is nonetheless true that *male peer support* is one of the most powerful determinants of why men use IPSV.

Originally labelled by me in 1988, the concept of male peer support refers to the attachments to male peers and the resources these men provide that encourage and legitimate woman abuse in intimate heterosexual relationships. A large body of empirical knowledge supports what Lee Bowker (1983) said nearly 34 years ago about all-male subcultures of violence:

> This is not a subculture that is confined to a single class, religion, occupational grouping, or race. It is spread throughout all parts of society. Men are socialized by other subculture members to accept common definitions of the situation, norms, values, and beliefs about male dominance and the necessity of keeping their wives in line. These violence-supporting social relations may occur at any time and in any place.
>
> (pp. 135–136)

Male peer pressure that perpetuates and rationalizes the sexual objectification of women and the sexual abuse of them is found within a wide variety of communities of all ethnicities and social classes. Such peer influence has been reported, to name a just a few, among African-American men in Chicago (Wilson, 1996), among Puerto Rican drug dealers in East Harlem, New York and poor African-American boys in parts of St. Louis (Bourgois, 1995; Miller, 2008), on Canadian college campuses and their immediate surroundings (DeKeseredy & Schwartz, 1998a), in rural Ohio and Kentucky (DeKeseredy

& Schwartz, 2009; Hall-Sanchez, 2014; Websdale, 1998), and in rural Australia, rural New Zealand, and rural South Africa (Campbell, 2000; Jewkes et al., 2006; Wendt, 2009). Pro-abuse male peer support groups also exist in cyberspace, and many men who sexually assault women consume and share electronic forms of pornography with their male friends (DeKeseredy & Corsianos, 2016; DeKeseredy & Olsson, 2011; DeKeseredy & Schwartz, 2013).

## What does male peer support look like?

Three types of male peer support consistently contribute to IPSV in a variety of intimate relationships: frequently drinking with male friends, informational support, and attachment to abusive peers. Informational support is the guidance and advice that influences men to abuse their current or former female partners, and attachment to abusive peers is having male friends who also abuse women. In addition to hunting with male peers, going to sporting events, and engaging in some other types of "leisure activities" (e.g., consuming Internet porn), frequently drinking with friends is often associated with the development of a particular kind of masculinity that objectifies women and endorses male behavior that endorses woman abuse. For example, one of the women who participated in Hall-Sanchez's (2014) study of separation/divorce sexual assault in rural Ohio stated:

> He would leave on Friday morning and return late Sunday. I would see him pack a few clothes but mostly beer, bullets, and porn. . . . I never understood how all that went together but he would tell me that they would drink, go scout the stuff and set up their spots in the woods, and come back to camp and drink, shoot targets, watch porn, guy talk, play cards, you know the usual guy stuff. They would tell dirty jokes and look at porn. . . . No women allowed and that is how they wanted it. That was a place where they could get away with demeaning women and get a pat on the back for "putting women in their place." I am sure all those guys did the same thing so it's no wonder Sundays were always bad for me.
>
> (p. 503)

Similarly, as is the case with college men who sexually abuse women, many of DeKeseredy and Schwartz's (2009) 43 rural Ohio female respondents reported that "nights out drinking with the boys" were contexts that often supported patriarchal conversations about women and how to control them. As one interviewee stated:

> Um, they're basically like him. They sit around, talk about women, and gossip. They're the biggest gossips there ever was. But they sit around and brag how many times they get it and how they keep their women in line, and you know, just like crap, you know.
>
> (p. 67)

There are several possible explanations for the relationship between sexual assault and frequently drinking with male friends. On one hand, men may be sexual aggressors in the first place and may drink heavily to relieve guilt. They may join groups of similarly like-minded men, who spend time convincing each other that they are right in sexually objectifying women and using alcohol heavily. On the other hand, the same data would support an explanation that men join a peer group, such as a fraternity, where they learn that such behaviors are, in fact, legitimate. At that point, they begin to act in that manner (Schwartz & DeKeseredy, 1997).

The social settings described above and by women interviewed by Hall-Sanchez (2014) and DeKeseredy and Schwartz (2009) are also examples of the factor of informational support, which is not restricted to group drinking events. For instance, the partner of one of DeKeseredy and Schwartz's interviewees spent much time with his cousin who "hated women" and who often called them "fuckin' bitches" and "whore sluts." Such language is certainly not limited to rural men. Many U.S. college men speak similarly while drinking and watching porn together (DeKeseredy & Corsianos, 2016). Kimmel (2008) frequently discovered that:

> They get angry. Each time I happened on a group of guys engaged in group pornography consumption, they spent a good deal of time jiving with each other about what they'd like to do to the girl on the screen, yelling at her, calling her a whore and a bitch and cheering on the several men who will proceed to penetrate her simultaneously.
>
> (p. 187)

Using pornographic videos to strengthen male "misogynist bonds" is not a relatively new phenomenon. Rather, it dates back to the 1890s (Slayden, 2010). Cinematic pornography originated in 16 mm silent films:

> usually shown in private all-male "smokers" in such contexts as bachelor parties and the like. Within such a context, the men laughed and joked and talk among themselves while watching the sexually explicit films about women, who though they were absent from the audience, were the likely butt of the jokes, laughing, and rude remarks.
>
> (Lehman, 2006, p. 4)

The contribution of pornography to IPSV is related to male peer support (see DeKeseredy, 2015 and Chapter 13). Further, numerous men learn to sexually objectify women through their consumption of porn (DeKeseredy & Corsianos, 2016; Jensen, 2007). Consider what Kimmel (2008) found in his study of "guys" (men between the ages of 16 and 26): "Guys tend to like to watch the extreme stuff, the double penetration and humiliating scenes; they watch it together in groups of guys, and they make fun of the women in the scene" (p. 181).

It is also well documented empirically that many college men belong to *hypererotic subcultures* in which members have high expectations of having sex and then end up feeling disappointed or angry if women reject their advances (DeKeseredy & Schwartz, 2013; Kanin, 1985). The type of informational support these men receive is learning from their peers to *expect* to engage in a very high level of consensual intercourse, or what to them is sexual conquest. The problem is that, for most men, such goals are impossible to achieve. When they fall short of what they see as their friends' high expectations, and perhaps short of what they believe their friends are all actually achieving, some of these men experience *relative deprivation*. This sexual frustration, caused by a "reference-group-anchored sex drive" can result in predatory sexual conduct (DeKeseredy & Corsianos, 2016; Kanin, 1967; Schwartz & DeKeseredy, 1997). The men are highly frustrated, not because they are deprived of sex in some objective sense, but because they feel inadequate or unable to engage in what they have defined as the proper amount of sex.

Since the late 1990s, Martin Schwartz and I (1998b) have continually argued that the sharing of cyber porn helps create and maintain patriarchal male peer groups. This sharing reinforces attitudes that reproduce and reconstitute ideologies of male dominance by approvingly depicting women as objects to be conquered and consumed (DeKeseredy & Corsianos, 2016; DeKeseredy & Schwartz, 2013). Such sharing also makes it difficult for users to separate sexual fantasy from reality and assists them in their attempts to initiate female victims and break down their resistance to sexual acts (Dines, 2010).

There is another type of online male peer support subculture that provides pro-ISPV informational support: anti-feminist men's rights activists (Dragiewicz, 2011). One case in point is the organization Return of Kings, led by Daryushi Valizadeh. This group has a growing following and holds public meetings that claim certain misogynistic acts are acceptable. Online articles written by Valizadeh and other members of Return of Kings assert that misogynists are better for women than feminists, that women should not be able to vote, that rape on private property should be legalized, that transgender women who have sexual relations with heterosexual men are rapists, and that women are biologically determined to follow the orders of men.

It is necessary to take anti-feminist online male peer support groups seriously. As Dragiewicz (2011) puts it, the use of men's rights sites "as places for like-minded men to seek out and receive peer support for violence-supportive attitudes is a serious concern for those interested in decreasing domestic violence, especially when we recognize their similarities to batterer accounts" (p. 137).

Turning now to attachments to abusive male peers, this factor plays a major role in a wide variety of contexts. Men with friends who physically, sexually, and emotionally abuse current and former female intimates are prone to the same behavior (DeKeseredy & Schwartz, 2013). Space limitations preclude all the studies supporting this claim and thus only one recent project is briefly reviewed here. Of the 43 rural Ohio women interviewed by me and Schwartz

(2009), 20 (47%) said that they knew their partners' friends also physically or sexually abused women. One interviewee said that *all* of her ex-partner's friends hit women or sexually assaulted them, and several women said they directly observed their partners' friends abusing female intimates. Jackie is one such participant: "I watched a friend of his who shoved a friend of mine up against a wall . . . and try to, you know, have his way with her" (p. 68). A few perpetrators enlisted the aid of their friends to sexually abuse some of these women. Such male peer support can involve forcing women to have sex with a man's friends, which is what happened to this person:

> Well, him and his friend got me so wasted. They took turns with me and I remembered most of it, but, um, there was also drugs involved. Not as much on my behalf as theirs. I was just drunk. And I did remember most of it, and the next morning I woke up feeling so dirty and degraded and then it ended up getting around that I was the slut. . . . And in my eyes that was rape, due to the fact that I was so drunk. And I definitely don't deserve that. And I was hurting. I was hurting the next day.
>
> (p. 68)

Several women in our sample who were forced to have group sex were also beaten after going through brutal degradation experiences. Lorraine recalled an incident that occurred during the end of her relationship: "He wanted me to have sex with a few people. Okay, like I was telling you earlier, and I didn't want to. . . . And, uh, I finally did. And then I got beat for it because I did. I tried not to, but then when we did, I got beat" (p. 70).

In South Africa, a version of this kind of gang rape is referred to as "streamlining." It is, according to Jewkes et al. (2006, p. 2951):

> essentially a rape by two or more perpetrators. It is an unambiguously defiling and humiliating act, and it is often a punishment, yet at the same time it is an act that is often regarded by its perpetrators as rooted in a sense of entitlement (Wood, 2005). A woman may be streamlined to punish her for having another partner; for behaving outside gender norms (e.g., when deeply intoxicated) (Wojcicki, 2002); for being successful; or for imagining she could be superior. Streamlining is sometimes an act of male bonding, a "favor" to the boyfriends' friends (Niehaus, 2005; Wood, 2005)

More research is needed on the male peer support dynamics covered here and elsewhere (e.g., DeKeseredy & Schwartz, 2013, 2015). However, as Dawn Currie (1995) put it 22 years ago, "Research alone does not result in social change. Social transformation is the consequence of a number of interrelated activities, which often require lobbying, the development of policy initiatives, consultation, etc." (p. 44).

## Challenging male peer support

The first step toward preventing the development of male peer support subcultures is to get more men to acknowledge that reducing IPSV is "men's work" (Messner, Greenberg, & Peretz, 2015). They need to recognize that this form of gendered violence is caused by men, and men are going to need to be involved in any solutions to it. Some excellent resources used to help achieve this goal are the practical writings of Jackson Katz (2006, 2015), Rus Funk (2006), Messner et al. (2015), and other feminist men (e.g., Fisher, 2011).

The above materials recommend feasible steps men can take to change their lives and those of others. They help get men involved in an ongoing process of changing themselves, self-examination, and self-discovery (DeKeseredy et al., 2000), with the ultimate goal of shedding their "patriarchal baggage" (Thorne-Finch, 1992). Though a relatively small, but growing group, these men work individually and collectively to change other men. Of course, staying within the level of micro dynamics (changing yourself or small groups) will do little to generate fundamental social transformation; critiquing the broader social and economic structure and institutions like the pornography industry, the military, the mainstream media, professional sports, and the justice system is also necessary.

Anti-violence men are scattered throughout the U.S., the U.K., Australia, Canada, and many other countries. Individually, they engage in strategies such as these, suggested by me and Schwartz (2013), Thorne-Finch (1992), the University of Kentucky's Violence Intervention and Prevention Center (2012), Warshaw (1988) and others (e.g., Funk, 2006):

- Put a sticker on your office door declaring your workplace a woman abuse-free zone.
- Confront male friends, classmates, co-workers, teachers, and others who make sexist jokes or who engage in sexist conversations.
- Confront the above people and others who speak about violent and dehumanizing pornography in an approving manner.
- Ask a woman in your life what you can do to help take a stand against violence.
- Have a conversation with a younger man or boy who looks up to you about how important it is for men to help end violence.
- Support and participate in woman abuse awareness programs.

Teaming up with other men to implement collective strategies is another vital step. A good place to start is to get involved with an organization, such as the White Ribbon Campaign. This international men's movement was initiated in Canada in October 1991 by the Men's Network for Change (MNC) in Toronto, Ottawa, London, Kingston, and Montreal in response to a mass shooting that occurred on December 6, 1989. That day, Marc Lepine shot and killed 14 female students at the University of Montreal, in what is now known as the Montreal Massacre. He repeatedly stated that he hated women and feminists, a sentiment shared by many serial and mass killers (DeKeseredy, Fabricius, & Hall-Sanchez, 2015).

> There are major advantages to working with groups such as the White Ribbon Campaign. One is that it helps men to "avoid reinventing the wheel" because, like many women involved in the struggle to end woman abuse, they are at risk of "burning out" or wasting their time and energy if they simply duplicate the work done by other progressive organizations (Thorne-Finch, 1992, p. 257)

The individual and collective efforts of such men can make a difference. Consider these indicators of success:

- Research shows that campaigns that encourage men to hold other men accountable for their abuse are likely to be effective, while those that indiscriminately blame all men are not.
- Male friends and relatives of women abusers can have a major impact on their behavior by addressing the abuse directly and defining it as unacceptable.
- Communicating with men about the importance of condemning abuse and providing them with some advice on how to confront abusers in a way that does not jeopardize their female partners will eventually create an environment in which woman abuse becomes socially unacceptable (DeKeseredy, 2011; DeKeseredy & MacLeod, 1997; Katz, 2015).

## References

Bourgois, P. (1995). *In search of respect: Selling crack in El Barrio*. New York, NY: Cambridge University Press.

Bowker, L.H. (1983). *Beating wife-beating*. Lexington, MA: Lexington Books.

Campbell, H. (2000). The glass phallus: Pub(lic) masculinity and drinking in rural New Zealand. *Rural Sociology, 65*, 532–536.

Currie, D.H. (1995). *Student safety at the University of British Columbia: Preliminary findings of a student safety study*. Vancouver, Canada: University of British Columbia.

DeKeseredy, W.S. (2011). *Violence against women: Myths, facts, controversies*. Toronto: University of Toronto Press.

DeKeseredy, W.S. (1988). Woman abuse in dating relationships: The relevance of social support theory. *Journal of Family Violence, 3*, 1–13.

DeKeseredy, W.S. (2011). *Violence against women: Myths, facts, controversies*. Toronto: University of Toronto Press.

DeKeseredy, W.S. (2015). Patriarchy.com: Adult Internet pornography and the abuse of women. In C.M. Renzetti & R. Kennedy Bergen (Eds.), *Understanding diversity: Celebrating difference, challenging inequality* (pp. 186–199). Boston, MA: Pearson.

DeKeseredy, W.S., & Corsianos, M. (2016). *Violence against women in pornography*. New York, NY: Routledge.

DeKeseredy, W.S., & MacLeod, L. (1997). *Woman abuse: A sociological story*. Toronto, Canada: Harcourt Brace.

DeKeseredy, W.S., & Olsson, P. (2011). Adult pornography, male peer support, and violence against women: The contribution of the "dark side" of the Internet. In M. Vargas Martin, M. Garcia-Ruiz, & A. Edwards (Eds.), *Technology for facilitating humanity and combating social deviations: Interdisciplinary perspectives* (pp. 34–50). Hershey, PA: IGI Global.

DeKeseredy, W.S., & Schwartz, M.D. (1998a). *Woman abuse on campus: Results from the Canadian national survey*. Thousand Oaks, CA: Sage.

DeKeseredy, W.S., & Schwartz, M.D. (1998b). Male peer support and woman abuse in postsecondary school courtship: Suggestions for new directions in sociological research. In R.K. Bergen (Ed.), *Issues in intimate violence* (pp. 83–96). Thousand Oaks, CA: Sage.

DeKeseredy, W.S., & Schwartz, M.D. (2009). *Dangerous exits: Escaping abusive relationships in rural America*. New Brunswick, NJ: Rutgers University Press.

DeKeseredy, W.S., & Schwartz, M.D. (2013). *Male peer support and violence against women: The history and verification of a theory*. Boston, MA: Northeastern University.

DeKeseredy, W.S., & Schwartz, M.D. (2015). Male peer support theory. In F.T. Cullen, P. Wilcox, J.L. Lux, & C. Lero Johnson (Eds.), *Sisters in crime revisited: Bringing gender into criminology* (pp. 302–322). New York, NY: Oxford University Press.

DeKeseredy, W.S., Schwartz, M.D., & Alvi, S. (2000). The role of profeminist men in dealing with woman abuse on the Canadian college campus. *Violence Against Women, 9*, 918–935.

DeKeseredy, W.S., Fabricius, A., & Hall-Sanchez, A. (2015). Fueling aggrieved entitlement: The contribution of women against feminism postings. In W.S. DeKeseredy & L. Leonard (Eds.), *Crimsoc report 4: Gender, victimology & restorative justice* (pp. 1–33). Hook, UK: Waterside Press.

Dines, G. (2010). *Pornland: How porn has hijacked our sexuality*. Boston, MA: Beacon Press.

Dragiewicz, M. (2011). *Equality with a vengeance: Men's rights groups, battered women, and antifeminist backlash*. Boston, MA: Northeastern University Press.

Fisher, S. (2011). *Male advocates for women's human rights handbook*. Suva, Fiji: Fiji Women's Crisis Center.

Funk, R.E. (2006). *Reaching men: Strategies for preventing sexist attitudes, behaviors, and violence*. Indianapolis, IN: Jist Life.

Hall-Sanchez, A.K. (2014). Male peer support, hunting, and separation/divorce sexual assault in rural Ohio. *Critical Criminology, 22*, 495–510.

Jensen, R. (2007). *Getting off: Pornography and the end of masculinity*. Cambridge, MA: South End Press.

Jewkes, R., Dunkle, K., Koss, M.P., Levin, J.B., Nduna, M., Jama, N., & Sikweyiya, Y. (2006). Rape perpetration by young rural South African men: Prevalence, patterns, and risk factors. *Social Science and Medicine, 63*, 2949–2961.

Kanin, E.J. (1967). An examination of sexual aggression as a response to sexual frustration. *Journal of Marriage and the Family, 29*, 428–433.

Kanin, E.J. (1985). Date rapists: Differential sexual socialization and relative deprivation. *Archives of Sexual Behavior, 14*, 219–231.

Katz, J. (2006). *The macho paradox: Why some men hurt women and how all men can help*. Naperville, IL: Sourcebooks.

Katz, J. (2015). Engaging men in the prevention of violence against women. In H. Johnson, B.S. Fisher, & V. Jaquier (Eds.), *Critical issues on violence against women: International perspectives and promising strategies* (pp. 233–243). London, UK: Routledge.

Kimmel, M. (2008). *Guyland: The perilous world where boys become men.* New York, NY: Harper.

Lehman, P. (2006). Introduction: "A dirty little secret" – Why teach and study pornography? In P. Lehman (Ed.), *Pornography: Film and culture* (pp. 1–24). New Brunswick, NJ: Rutgers University Press.

Messner, M.A., Greenberg, M.A., & Peretz, T. (2015). *Some men: Feminist allies & the movement to end violence against women.* New York, NY: Oxford University Press.

Miller, J. (2008). *Getting played: African-American girls, urban inequality, and gendered violence.* New York, NY: New York University Press.

Niehaus, I. (2005). Masculine dominance in sexual violence: Interpreting accounts of three cases of rape in the South Africa Lowveld. In G. Reid & L. Walker (Eds.), *Men behaving differently* (pp. 65–83). Cape Town, South Africa: Juta.

Schwartz, M.D, & DeKeseredy, W.S. (1997). *Sexual assault on the college campus: The role of male peer support.* Thousand Oaks, CA: Sage.

Slayden, D. (2010). Debbie does Dallas again and again: Pornography, technology, and market innovation. In F. Attwood (Eds.), *Porn.com: Making sense of online pornography* (pp. 54–68). New York, NY: Peter Lang.

Thorne-Finch, R. (1992). *Ending the silence: The origins and treatment of male violence against men.* Toronto, Canada: University of Toronto Press.

True, J. (2012). *The political economy of violence against women.* New York, NY: Oxford University Press.

University of Kentucky Violence Intervention and Prevention Center (2012). Green dots for men. Retrieved from: www.uky.edu/StudentAffairs/VIPCenter/learn_greendot.php.

Warshaw, R. (1988). *I never called it rape.* New York, NY: Harper & Row.

Websdale, R. (1998). *Rural woman battering and the justice system: An ethnography.* Thousand Oaks, CA: Sage.

Wendt, S. (2009). *Domestic violence in rural Australia.* Annandale, Australia: The Federation Press.

Wilson, W.J. (1996). *When work disappears: The world of the new urban poor.* New York, NY: Knopf.

Wojcicki, J. (2002). "She drank his money": Survival sex and the problem of violence in taverns in Gauteng Province, South Africa. *Medical Anthropology, 16,* 267–293.

Wood, K. (2005). Contextualizing group rape in post-apartheid South Africa. *Culture, Health, and Sexuality, 7,* 303–317.

# Chapter 13

# The role of adult pornography in intimate partner sexual violence perpetrators' offending

*Walter S. DeKeseredy and Rus Ervin Funk*

## Introduction

This chapter is one of a rapidly growing number of scholarly articles, book chapters, and monographs that treat adult pornography and its negative effects as both major social problems and subjects worthy of in-depth scholarly inquiry. The main objective of our contribution is twofold: (1) to briefly review the research on the association between pornography and intimate partner sexual violence (IPSV), and (2) to recommend some strategies that educators and advocates can use to help reduce men's consumption of porn and the myriad of harms caused by such media.

## Definition of adult pornography

Not to be confused with erotica, which is "sexually suggestive or arousing material that is free of sexism, racism, and homophobia and is respectful of all human beings and animals portrayed" (Russell, 1993, p. 3), pornography is harmful on numerous levels. Women and men are represented in many different ways in pornography, but two things nearly all heterosexual pornographic images and writings have in common is that females are characterized as subordinate to males and the primary role is the provision of sex to men.

Adult pornography has significantly changed over the past few decades due to the Internet. Much, if not most, of it today is "gonzo – that genre which is all over the Internet and is today one of the biggest money-makers for the industry – which depicts hard core, body-punishing sex in which women are demeaned and debased" (Dines, 2010, p. xi). A common feature of contemporary porn videos is painful anal penetration as well as brutal gang rape and men slapping or choking women or pulling their hair while they penetrate them orally, vaginally, and anally (DeKeseredy, 2015a).

Such images are part and parcel of today's adult Internet pornography, but violent sexual images are available elsewhere. For instance, Bridges, Wosnitzer, Scharrer, Sun, and Liberman (2010) examined 304 scenes in 50 of the then most popular pornographic DVDs and found that nearly 90% contained physical aggression (mainly spanking, gagging, and slapping) and roughly 50% included verbal aggression, primarily name-calling. Males constituted most of the perpetrators and the targets of their physical and verbal aggression were "overwhelmingly female." Moreover, female targets often appeared to show pleasure or responded neutrally to male aggression. To make matters worse, as the porn industry grows and attracts an ever-growing consumer base, it is generating even more violent materials featuring demeaning and dehumanizing behaviors never before seen (DeKeseredy & Corsianos, 2016). It is not only anti-porn scholars and activists who assert that violent sex is now a normal part of the industry. Even porn producers publicly admit that it is the status quo (Abowitz, 2013; Dines, 2010).

As well, racism is a central element of some of today's pornography. Consider the following titles of videos uncovered by DeKeseredy (2015b) during a Google search using the words "racist porn" on September 3, 2014. His hunt generated 22 million results in 0.40 seconds and one salient example of the titles listed is *Racist bitch is forced to have sex with a black man*. Actually, many of the racist videos offer stereotypical images of the "sexually primitive black male stud" (Jensen, 2007, p. 66). Certainly, men and women of color are not the only people to be racially exploited by the porn industry. Keep in mind these films featured on the widely used site Xvideos.com: *Sexy latina rides a black bull in front of her husband* and *Me so Asian*.

Whether or not researchers ever obtain an absolutely accurate estimate of the percentage of people who consume adult pornography, most leading experts on the topic agree with Robert Jensen's contention that "It's become almost as common as comic books were for you and me" (cited in Gillespie, 2008, p. 3). In fact, studies of youth show that almost all boys in Northern Europe have at some point in their lives been exposed to pornography and 42% of Internet users ages 10 to 17 in the U.S. had viewed cyberporn (Hammaren & Johansson, 2007; Mossige, Ainsaar, & Svedin, 2007; Wolak, Mitchell, & Finkelhor, 2007).

Pornography consumers, by and large, are not innocent users who accidentally come across sexually explicit images, voices and texts. Nor are they constantly bombarded with such material. Rather, they tend to make a conscious effort to consume and distribute porn, and many consumers use it to inform their sexual attitudes and behaviors, some of which involve sexually assaulting current or former female partners (DeKeseredy & Schwartz, 2013).

## Pornography and IPSV

### Understanding the connection

Large and small surveys conducted in Canada and the U.S. between the late 1980s and late 1990s uncovered a sizable portion of women who have experienced pornography-related sexual and physical abuse in intimate adult relationships (DeKeseredy & Schwartz, 1998; Harmon & Check, 1989; Russell, 1990). The correlation between pornography and sexual assault is not restricted to North America. In Italy, for instance, one study of high school students uncovered strong associations between sexually harassing or raping peers and porn consumption (Bonino, Ciairano, Rabaglietti, & Cattelino, 2006). Another Italian survey of high school students found that females exposed to psychological violence committed by family members and to sexual violence by any type of perpetrator were significantly more likely to watch porn, especially violent porn, than females who were not exposed to such abuse. The researchers suggest a variety of possible reasons, ranging from the traumatic impact of sexual victimization to possible exposure to pornography as a concomitant of other risk factors involved in sexual abuse (Romito & Beltramini, 2011). In Sweden, a study of 1,933 boys uncovered a higher rate of violent porn use among those who reported sexually coercing someone compared to nondelinquent youth (Kjellgren, Priebe, Svedin, & Langstrom, 2012).

The bulk of other empirical work on adults' experiences with porn and IPSV involved gathering data from rape crisis workers who conducted phone and face-to-face interviews with sexual and physical assault survivors (Bergen & Bogle, 2000; Shope, 2004; Simmons, Lehmann, & Collier-Tennison, 2008). Collectively, this research reveals a strong linkage between men's porn consumption and female victimization. For example, Shope (2004) found that an abuser's use of porn doubled the risk of a physically assaulted woman being sexually assaulted.

More recently, using face-to-face interviews with 55 rural southeast Ohio women who were sexually abused during the period when they wanted to or were trying to end a relationship with a husband or live-in partner, or where such a relationship had already ended, DeKeseredy and Hall-Sanchez (2016) uncovered that 34 of their interviewees experienced porn-related sexual abuse. They also identify five significant themes related to men's porn consumption and their use of IPSV.

### Learning about sex through pornography

"Candace" highlights the first theme, learning about sex through pornography, experienced by three women in the sample:

> I met a guy one time out West that I had a sexual experience with that was extremely rough and afterwards he had told me that no one had ever talked to him about sex. He learned from pornography. And so he shaved his balls because he didn't know it was, I mean I know a lot of people do. Someone is learning from porno as an educational thing?

### Comparison and imitation

Some studies, most of them conducted from the early 1980s to the late 1990s (see DeKeseredy & Corsianos, 2016), show that many women have been harmed or upset by their partners' requests or demands to imitate pornographic scenarios, underscoring DeKeseredy and Hall-Sanchez's second theme: comparison and imitation. Consider Alison's experience. Her ex-partner viewed violent porn and she describes the familiar language and demeaning behaviors often featured in gonzo videos:

> I remember him making me give him oral sex and holding me by the hair and I don't remember if it was after a fight or what. He's done that I don't know how many times. He used to urinate on me and then want sex, I mean after getting hit and stuff. . . . He would talk the whole time he was doing that and saying things like uh, "you're my bitch" or "you like it bitch don't you." And stuff like that. Um, "this is my ass, you know I'll kill for my ass." Stuff like that and it would be just as violent as the beating and basically you just lay there and let it happen.

### The introduction of other sexual partners

In total, seven women reported the third theme identified – the introduction of other sexual partners. Below is Silvia's experience:

> He had ended up being with a man and he would make me watch . . . When he wanted sex in a group thing or with his buddies or made me have sex with a friend of his. See one time he made me have sex with a friend of his for him to watch, then he got mad and hit me afterwards. And I didn't quite understand why he got mad.

### Surreptitious videotaping

Cara is one of four women who was unknowingly videotaped during consensual and nonconsensual sex – the fourth theme. Her ex-partner used alcohol to try to "loosen" her up and to make her try new sexual positions. This incident prompted her to leave him:

> When I woke up there was like a light on me. He works at the TV station here. . . . Anyways, um, he was videotaping it . . . and that was it, I said this has got to end. And he still carries the video tape around to this day. I have yet to view it.

Denise's ex-husband uses a videotape of a sexual assault to maintain control over her, even after their separation:

He ended up tying me up and blindfolding me and then, without my knowledge, videotaped it. And then after we had split up for good, he left the tape on Bill's car that was at my house and a letter with it saying that it was spread all over town. I contacted the police department and they wanted to watch the tape and I wouldn't give it to them. And then the officer that responded to it called his wife and told her, because this town is a small community and everybody knows everybody and I used to work there. He called and told her and she went and told my best friend because they are neighbors.

### The overall culture of pornography

Turning to the last theme, the overall culture of pornography, DeKeseredy and Hall-Sanchez uncovered various nuanced reports from five interviewees about how the broader pornographic culture affects women's lives. Billie's ex-partner, for example, "wasn't really into porn" that she knew of, but throughout the course of her interview, she strived to make sense of his fetishes that ultimately played a major role in her sexually abusive experiences:

He had a few particular fetishes. And uh, you know at first I thought it was okay but then it became really uncomfortable but he wasn't you know, wasn't willing to change that. And I guess maybe a part of me still loved him and maybe wanted to, you know, please him, but it was just, you know, perverse to me. It was like it went against the grain of everything I ever held, however I ever looked at sex and how it was supposed to be in a relationship. Um, so, but like I said, I mean, I was a completely different person. He totally changed me. It was all an emotional, physical, spiritual thing. It was all twisted up so it is really hard to explain . . . . And, also like, and he was kind of like a masochist type. . . . He became the sadist.

Eliminating pornography might not have an effect on these men's violent conduct. Yet, there is no doubt that the data presented here and elsewhere demonstrate that pornographic media are a major component of the problem of IPSV and other variants of woman abuse. We also know that, like violence against women, pornography is deeply entrenched in our society. How could it be such a lucrative business if only a small number of people used it (Lehman, 2006)? Moreover, we know that pornography consumption has a major impact on men's attitudes, beliefs, values, and, in many cases, their behavior. The "script" of heterosexual pornography is hostile to men's expression of empathy with their female sexual partners (Dines, Jensen, & Russo, 1998; Funk, 2004; Jensen, 2007), and some violent men use pornography as a "training manual for abuse" (Bergen & Bogle, 2000, p. 231). Certainly, many of the men who abused the women interviewed by DeKeseredy and Hall-Sanchez (2016) were graduates of what Bancroft (2002) refers to as "the Pornography School of Sexuality" (p. 185).

## Intervention and prevention strategies

### Working with perpetrators

Given the extent to which pornography is used by male IPSV offenders, it seems a minimal recommendation that all IPSV practitioners screen perpetrators for pornography consumption. However, doing what is minimalist is not enough; a much more thorough approach is necessary. An integral part of this comprehensive approach should first include complete prohibition of pornography consumption for perpetrators while in intervention. The Association of Treatment for Sex Abusers (ATSA) establishes this as a standard for treatment programs with adolescent and adult sex abusers. It is an appropriate baseline because IPSV perpetrators receive treatment or intervention in varied contexts. Practitioners working with female survivors of other types of intimate violence should, as part of their screening process, also universally explore for patterns of pornography use.

As a part of their treatment, perpetrators need a way to examine the connection between their pornography use, their sexist attitudes, and their sexually abusive behaviors. The continuum of harm exercise is one effective way of achieving this goal (Funk, 2014). Presented in Box 13.1, practitioners should put this continuum on a flip chart or white board.

### Widening our focus

Space limitations preclude a detailed exploration of other activities and strategies that practitioners can use to integrate a critical examination of pornography into intervention with male IPSV offenders. However, we would be remiss if we did not briefly address the importance of working more broadly because male pornography use has reached the point of being both normal and normalized in our society. Consider that the average age in which males start consuming Internet porn is 11 (DeKeseredy & Corsianos, 2016; Dines, 2010). Pornography consumption should be viewed as a social problem requiring social strategies to curb. Educating men in general about the harms of pornography use and working for broader social change are critical factors that will, if done in concert, ultimately increase the effectiveness of individual-level intervention with male IPSV offenders.

These efforts can help provide an atmosphere in which men show respect for each other and change attitudes, increase knowledge, and change behavioral intentions (DeKeseredy & Schwartz, 2013). One example of this kind of social change effort (which focuses on adolescents) is the film *In the Picture*. Developed in Australia by Maree Crabbe as part of the Brophy Family and Youth Services'

---

### Box 13.1 The continuum of harm

**Less harmful**                                              **Most harmful**

◄─────────────────────────────────────────────────────────►

Offenders need to locate the following behaviors on the continuum in relation to the other behaviors and to identify the degree of harm inherent in each behavior:

- View women I meet as a body part.
- View my partner as her sexual body part(s).
- Prostituting my partner.
- Prostituting my daughter or son.
- Participating in bachelor parties where women are dancing naked.
- Participating in a party where women are dancing naked and then are prostituted (such as drawing to see who gets a blow job).
- Look at porn sites that advertise "young girls."
- Using language with other men about women's body parts and what we would like do to them.
- My 8-year-old son comes across pornography while searching for a Mario Brothers Game.
- My 10-year old daughter comes across pornography while searching for a Mario Brothers Game.
- Showing my 11-year-old son pornography.
- Showing my 13-year-old son pornography.
- Showing my 16-year-old son pornography.
- Showing my 21-year-old son pornography.
- Paid for a woman to have sex with my son.
- Watched bestiality porn.
- Watched rape porn.
- Watched snuff porn.

---

community education project *Reality & Risk: Pornography, Young People and Sexuality, In the Picture* comes on a DVD and has 82 resources designed to comprehensively address the issues of explicit sexual imagery that many of our youth are encountering on a regular basis.

We run the risk of forever treating the survivors and perpetrators of IPSV if we do not change patriarchal social norms and move more aggressively toward prevention. One of our key efforts should be helping boys and men develop what Michael Kimmel (2008) coins as a "new model of masculinity":

Young men must understand on a deep level that being a real man isn't going along with what you know in your heart to be cruel, inhumane, stupid, humiliating, and dangerous. Being a real man means doing the right thing, standing up to immorality and injustice when you see it, and expressing compassion, not contempt, for those who are less fortunate. In other words, it's about being courageous. So much of Guyland encourages cowardice – being a passive bystander, going along with what seems to be the crowd's consensus.

(p. 287)

## Conclusion

Pornography is poisoning our society on many levels, including contributing to IPSV. Addressing this issue requires a multidimensional approach. One or two methods alone will not succeed. The work involved in confronting pornography is destined to be ongoing and ever-changing, as will be the porn industry and its collaborators' resistance to attempts to eliminate degrading, violent, and racist sexual media. As Jensen (2007) puts it, those who want to end the pornification of our society "have a lot of work to do" (p. 184). What we and many others believe are effective means of doing so are suggested in this chapter, but there are, of course, many more initiatives that could be proposed and have been by others (e.g., DeKeseredy & Corsianos, 2016). The ultimate goal is for all of us, whatever role we play, to get involved in community-based efforts to curb pornography and IPSV.

## References

Abowitz, R. (2013, April 21). Rob Black, porn's dirty whistleblower, spills trade secrets. *The Daily Beast*. Retrieved from: www.thedailybeast.com/articles/2013/04/21/rob-black-porn-s-dirty-whistlebower-spills-trade-secrets.html.

Bancroft, L. (2002). *Why does he do that? Inside the minds of angry and controlling men*. New York, NY: Berkley.

Bergen, R.K., & Bogle, K.A. (2000). Exploring the connection between pornography and sexual violence. *Violence and Victims, 15*, 227–234.

Bonino, S., Ciairano, S., Rabaglietti, E., & Cattelino, E. (2006). Use of pornography and self-reported engagement in sexual violence among adolescents. *European Journal of Developmental Psychology, 3*, 265–288.

Bridges, A.J., Wosnitzer, R., Scharrer, E., Sun, C., & Liberman, R. (2010). Aggression and sexual behavior in best-selling pornography videos: A content analysis. *Violence Against Women, 16*, 1065–1085.

DeKeseredy, W.S. (2015a). Patriarchy.com: Adult Internet pornography and the abuse of women. In C.M. Renzetti & R. Kennedy Bergen (Eds.), *Understanding diversity: Celebrating difference, challenging inequality* (pp. 186–199). Boston, MA: Pearson.

DeKeseredy, W.S. (2015b). Critical criminological understandings of adult pornography and woman abuse: New progressive directions in research and theory. *International Journal for Crime, Justice and Social Democracy, 4*, 4–21.

DeKeseredy, W.S., & Corsianos, M. (2016). *Violence against women in pornography*. London, UK: Routledge.

DeKeseredy, W.S., & Hall-Sanchez, A. (2016). Adult pornography and violence against women in the heartland: Results from a rural southeast Ohio study. *Violence Against Women*. Advance online publication. doi: 10.1177/1077801216648795.

DeKeseredy, W.S., & Schwartz, M.D. (1998). *Woman abuse on campus: Results from the Canadian national survey*. Thousand Oaks, CA: Sage.

DeKeseredy, W.S., & Schwartz, M.D. (2013). *Male peer support and violence against women: The history and verification of a theory*. Boston, MA: Northeastern University Press.

Dines, G. (2010). *Pornland: How porn has hijacked our sexuality*. Boston, MA: Beacon Press.

Dines, G., Jensen, R., & Russon, A. (Eds.) (1998). *Pornography: The production and consumption of inequality*. New York, NY: Routledge.

Funk, R.E. (2004). What does pornography say about me(n)?: How I became an anti-pornography activist. In C. Stark & R. Whisnant (Eds.), *Not for sale: Feminists resisting prostitution and pornography* (pp. 331–351). Melbourne, Australia: Spinifex Press.

Funk, R. E. (2014). *What's wrong with this picture?: Examining the harms of viewing pornography and the links to men's perpetration of gender based violence*. Louisville, KY: MensWork.

Gillespie, I. (2008, June 11). Nowadays, it's brutal, accessible; pornography. *London Free Press*, A3.

Hammaren, N., & Johansson, T. (2007). Hegemonic masculinity and pornography: Young people's attitudes toward and relations to pornography. *Journal of Men's Studies*, 15, 57–71.

Harmon, P.A., & Check, J.V. P. (1989). *The role of pornography in woman abuse*. Toronto, Canada: LaMarsh Research Program on Violence and Conflict Resolution, York University.

Jensen, R. (2007). *Getting off: Pornography and the end of masculinity*. Cambridge, MA: South End Press.

Kimmel, M. (2008). *Guyland: The perilous world where boys become men*. New York, NY: Harper.

Kjellgren, C., Priebe, G., Svedin, C. G., Mossige, S., & Langstrom, N. (2012). Female youth who sexually coerce: Prevalence, risk, and protective factors in two national high school surveys. *Journal of Sex Medicine*, 8, 3354–3362.

Lehman, P. (2006). Introduction: "A dirty little secret": Why teach and study pornography? In P. Lehman (Ed.), *Pornography: Film and culture* (pp. 1–24). New Brunswick, NJ: Rutgers University Press.

Mossige, S., Ainsaar, M., & Svedin, C. (Eds.). (2007). *The Baltic Sea regional study on adolescent sexuality* (NOVA Rapport 18/07). Oslo, Norway: Norwegian Social Research.

Romita, P., & Beltramini, L. (2011). Watching pornography: Gender differences, violence and victimization. An exploratory study in Italy. *Violence Against Women*, 17(10), 1313–1326. doi 10.1177/1077801211424555.

Russell, D. (1990). *Rape in marriage* (2nd ed.). Bloomington, IN: Indiana University Press.

Russell, D. (1993). *Against pornography: The evidence of harm*. Berkeley, CA: Russell Publications.

Shope, J.H. (2004). When words are not enough: The search for the effect of pornography on abused women. *Violence Against Women*, 10(1), 56–72.

Simmons, C.A., Lehmann, P., & Collier-Tenison, S. (2008). Linking male use of the sex industry to controlling behaviors in violent relationships: An exploratory analysis. *Violence Against Women*, 14(4), 406–417.

Wolak, J., Mitchell, K.J., & Finkelhor, D. (2007). Unwanted and wanted exposure to online pornography in a national sample of youth Internet users. *Pediatrics*, 119, 247–255.

## Chapter 14

# The court's response to intmate partner sexual violence perpetrators

*Anna Carline and Patricia Easteal*

## Introduction

Any efforts to change the way IPSV defendants are treated need to recognize that the courts' responses do not take place in a vacuum, but are embedded within the attitudes held by many in the community and by the legacy of legal precedent and past practice. The "license to rape" (the spousal exemption from sexual assault charges), although now abolished in most countries, continues to have a potent impact on the beliefs and actions of the courts and the community (Carline & Easteal, 2014). If you work in the criminal justice system it is useful for you to learn more about why this is so. In this chapter, we will highlight some of the ways that the legacy of the fiction ripples into the courtroom. We provide several examples of how IPSV continues not to be seen as "real rape" and how this affects the legal response to perpetrators. We also include a few recommendations. Some are relevant for those who work in the Courts. Other suggestions are more relevant for readers who are advocates or in positions to work toward law reform and/or policy changes.

## Not quite "real" rape

Since the 1980s, studies of attitudes toward partner rape have found that some people simply do not believe that husbands ever use force to compel their wives to have sex; some believe it's rare; some believe wives have no right to say no; and many do not think this type of sexual assault harms the victim because she is used to having consensual sex with her abuser (Basile, 2002; Ferro, Cermele, & Saltzman, 2008). A mythology persists which constructs marital rape as less damaging or injurious than other types of rape (Easteal, 2001; Edwards, Turchik, Dardis, Reynolds, & Gidycz, 2011). Be aware that within the criminal justice system, the same minimization of the harm of IPSV and reduced culpability of the offender is reflected (Carline & Easteal, 2014). As stated in an Australian appeals matter, IPSV may be seen as "quite different from the characteristics of the more usual cases of non-consensual sexual intercourse which come before the Courts" (*Turnell v The Queen* [2006] NSWCCA 399, [65]).

For example, note that the high rate of prosecutorial discontinuances in all sexual assault cases is slightly higher in partner rape (Heenan, 2004a; Lea, Lanvers, & Shaw, 2003). Evidently, prosecutors are influenced either consciously or unconsciously by the continuum of "real" rape and will "run" with the cases that they believe will result in a conviction. For instance, in Canada, despite the abolition of the marital rape exemption in 1983, "both Crown and defence counsel generally translated wife/partner rape as 'bad sex' or 'unwanted sex' but not *really* as rape" (Lazar, 2010, p. 333).

Further concern regarding prosecutorial decision-making stems from the English case of *R v A* ([2012] EWCA Crim 434). The defendant in this case was an IPSV victim who was convicted for perverting the course of justice after she falsely retracted an allegation of rape against her abusive husband. Despite acknowledging the psychological impact of the domestic abuse suffered, as well as the pressure the perpetrator and his sister placed on her to retract the complaint, the Court of Appeal upheld the conviction. Nevertheless, as Hoyano (2013) argues, the decision to prosecute an IPSV victim for a false retraction fundamentally undermines the legitimacy and integrity of the criminal justice system. It may also negatively impact rates of reporting, as women fear being prosecuted if they retract a complaint (which is not an uncommon feature of IPSV). The Director of Public Prosecutions has since developed a policy to deal with false retractions in rape and domestic violence cases which, if it had been applied in *R v A*, would have resulted in no further action. However, as Hoyano (2013, p. 245) notes, this is "unlikely to completely allay [any] apprehension," as the possibility of being prosecuted remains.

### Recommendation: Use expert witnesses

One way of assisting the court to understand the specific effects and harms of partner rape is to have expert testimony and/or reports by people who work in the area of violence against women as a normative part of the trial process. These experts may provide judges and jurors with the necessary information to better understand how IPSV is "real" rape. As demonstrated by Long (2007), their evidence might combat the myths about domestic violence and sexual assault, and how the mythology may intersect in the perception of IPSV.

### How consent is negated in IPSV and may not be understood

Consent is a complex legal construct. Therefore, it is essential to be aware that establishing the two elements of the offense of sexual assault is challenging, and that these problems seem to be magnified in the context of IPSV (Carline & Easteal, 2014). Unsurprisingly in a partner context, proving that the woman did not consent (a physical element) or an absence of consent that the defendant knew of, but chose to ignore (the fault element) is difficult, because of the history of consensual intercourse. This can problematically lead to the imposition of informal "presumed consent" or "continuing consent" models, even in jurisdictions such as Canada, which on the surface require affirmative consent (Lazar, 2010).

In a 2009 Australian judgment, for example, the judge indicated that defense *Counsel* in the final address had focused on the defendant's knowledge of lack of consent and had asked the jury to take into account the fact that the complainant and the appellant were married; that they had been living together for 15 years and *"how married couples might relate to each other in a sexual environment"* (*TK v R* (2009) 74 NSWLR 299, 328).

Understanding that no consent was given is made more problematic by survivors' experience of the different types of coercion: social, interpersonal, threat of physical force, and physical force (Finkelhor and Yllo, 1985). Many IPSV survivors experience multiple types of coercion both concurrently and over time, in the context of changing abuse patterns (Mahoney & Williams, 1998). Yet, we must emphasize that the legal interpretation of consent and its negation focuses far more upon physical force and injury, as illustrated in the sentencing remarks in a 2013 Australian Capital Territory case (*R v TN* [2013] ACT SC 64 (10 September 2013). Justice Penfold noted bruising, four loose teeth, swollen lips, and abrasions as a result of the attack. In sentencing the offender to almost five years of incarceration for raping his estranged wife of 22 years, she stated: "This was a particularly nasty sexual assault in the sense that it appears to have involved [the man] using a sexual violation to assert his power over his wife."

### Recommendation: Work to amend consent provisions or their interpretation

Expert witnesses and/or expert reports could be employed to explain what types of behavior are coercive and what could constitute negation of consent from the victim's perspective. Further law reform might help too. Pertinent provisions could be amended to state that consent is not relevant when actual bodily harm is involved. In cases of assault, and even indecent assault, the courts have affirmed that view. There is also precedent within rape common law. In the Canadian case of *R v Welsh* (1995) 86 OAC 200, it was held that a person cannot consent to a sexual act causing bodily harm.

Vitiation of consent could be defined more broadly to include the type of intimidation that can be generated in a marital type of relationship. As the Australian Law Reform Commission (2010, p. 1158) recommended, all jurisdictions should include that consent is negated if there is "abuse of a position 'of authority *or trust*'; and to threats against the 'complainant *or any other person*.'"

As an alternative to defining, or redefining, consent, attention has been given to the development of offenses in which the notion of consent is not so pivotal (Tadros, 2006). Such an approach, for example, has been adopted by some of those jurisdictions such as Michigan that operate a gradation scheme in which the law stipulates that in certain circumstances sexual activity is an offense, such as if the defendant is armed with a weapon, causes personal injury, or uses force or coercion (Mich Comp Laws § 750–520b(1) (1974). By focusing more on the violence used, as opposed to the sexual activity, the law recognizes that rape/sexual assault is fundamentally a crime of violence. Further, the prosecution does not have to prove the absence of consent. The focus is on the conduct of the defendant, as opposed to the complainant.

## Evidentiary barriers with IPSV

Be aware that a higher evidential threshold may be set in IPSV cases and, as Sack (2009, p. 937) notes, such differential treatment "demonstrates ongoing toleration for the view that married women are not entitled to legal autonomy." Additional evidentiary issues could include the disappearance of evidence, which can be used against the woman in court to further discredit her as a witness. Prompt disclosure and reporting are not the norm with this type of rape (Easteal & McOrmond-Plummer, 2006).

The admissibility or inadmissibility of prior violence evidence is extremely important too. From the perspective of the IPSV victim, *fear* of physical force may be the source of coercion. If testimony concerning family violence antecedents is not admitted and the incident is looked at in isolation from prior abuse, then the threat of force that vitiates or negates the victim's consent may not be understood.

Another problem concerns defense barristers' questioning of the victim witness about specific sexual activities between her and the accused. The aim is to suggest that "consensual sex was more likely to have occurred on the occasion in question, just as it had in the past" (Heenan, 2004a, p. 8). Although laws have been enacted to restrict the admission of previous sexual activity between the accused and the complainant in most Western countries, such provisions continue to be susceptible to problematic judicial interpretation in IPSV cases (Carline and Easteal, 2014). In the English House of Lords in *R v A (No 2* [2002] 1 AC 45) for instance, the Court maintained that previous sexual activity between the accused and the complainant was relevant to the issue of consent and therefore should be more readily admissible. And, across the world in Australia, the conviction in *Taylor v The Queen* [2009] NSWCCA 180 was quashed and "a miscarriage of justice" declared since "this is a case where the jury's view of ABC's credibility in her account of how the assault took place is of great importance." The crux of the appeal was that evidence about a continuing sexual relationship had not been admitted.

The underlying reasoning in these and other such cases appears to not recognize that consent is given anew each time and is a "decision," as opposed to "an emotion or a mind-set" (Ellison, 2010, p. 208). By implying that due to her previous sexual activity a woman is more likely to consent to sexual intercourse, there is an "inference that women are less likely to be raped by their sexual partners rather than others" (Boyle & MacCrimmon, 1998, p. 229). This may restrict these women's right to legal protection (Firth, 2006).

### Recommendation: Work for reform and judicial education that changes (interpretation of) the rules of evidence

Under most legislation, evidence is considered as relevant and therefore admitted if it "could rationally affect (directly or indirectly) the assessment of the probability of the existence of a *fact in issue* in the proceeding" (*Evidence Act 1995* (Cth) section 55). Judicial education about IPSV is required. To understand how consent is vitiated or negated, which is the *fact in issue,* judges must learn that IPSV should be seen within the dynamics and context of the other manifestations of family violence.

As far as evidence concerning previous sexual activities between the accused and the victim, McGlynn (2010, p. 225), in her feminist rewriting of *R v A (No 2),* suggests that the more discretionary Canadian *Criminal Code* s 276 could be adopted in other countries. In Canada, when sexual history evidence is admitted because it is deemed relevant to some other issue in the trial, the judge must warn the jury not to draw inappropriate inferences regarding consent and credibility (*R v Seaboyer* [1991] 2 SCR 577, 636). Although such judicial warnings regarding inappropriate inferences may have little effect (Schuller & Hastings, 2002; Schuller & Klippenstine, 2004), we believe their use is of value as they involve judicial officers challenging problematic assumptions regarding rape and consent.

Further to this, a significant online resource for judicial education regarding the nature and impact of IPSV has been developed in the U.S. by the National Judicial Education Program of Legal Momentum, *Intimate Partner Sexual Abuse: Adjudicating this Hidden Dimension of Domestic Violence Cases,* www.njep-ipsacourse.org. This free online course may be of use not only in relation to the development of appropriate judicial warnings, but also for professionals in all disciplines to extend their learning about IPSV.

## Legacies in sentencing

Instead of considering the violation of the trust in an intimate relationship as an aggravating factor, the judicial tendency may be the opposite: seeing the (previous) relationship as mitigating the sentence. For example, Easteal and Gani (2005) identified IPSV cases with histories of domestic violence in which judges considered offenders' emotional upset at a relationship breakup to be a mitigating variable at sentencing. If the woman has willingly had sex with the rapist at some point in the recent past, this may affect the judge's construction of the offense, perhaps viewing the defendant as having a genuine but unreasonable belief in consent. This is exemplified in the lenient sentences and

language used by some Australian judges (Easteal & Gani, 2005). The harm of
rape by a stranger often seems to be considered as relatively greater:

> The case was not one where a victim walking through a lonely street or
> park at night is seized by a complete stranger about whom she knows
> nothing and who, for all the victim knows, may well kill her when the
> intercourse is . . .
>
> (*Boney v R* [2008] NSWCCA 165)

> an extremely serious example of the offence of rape . . . She was unknown
> to you, taken from the street *where she had the right to feel safe*. She was
> attacked without explanation and suffered extremely serious injuries.
>
> (*R v Gill* [2008] VCC 0027, 46–47)

In Scotland, too, at least some judges still accept that a domestic relationship
operates in mitigation:

> Whilst the element of breach of trust involved in any domestic assault is
> an important factor in determining penalty, the significance of an ongoing
> sexual relationship in determining the penalty in a case such as this where
> the gravest feature is that there was penile penetration and the conviction
> is for rape, is a much more complex issue. The fact of the relationship is
> one of a complex host of facts and circumstances that have to be taken
> into account in determining appropriate sentence. In this case we consider
> that the trial judge gave insufficient weight to the fact that the couple had
> regularly engaged in sexual intercourse over a period of two years up to
> the night of the offence.
>
> (*HM Advocate v Petrie* [2011] HCJAC 1, [7])

In England and Wales, the sentencing of IPSV has evolved over the years.
Guidance was initially produced by the Court of Appeal in *R v Millberry* ([2003]
2 All ER 939), which was incorporated into the Sentencing Council's 2007
Definitive Guideline, and remained in force until April 2014. The court
agreed with a proposition from Sentencing Advisory Panel, regarding the
equal seriousness of relationship, acquaintance, and stranger rape. This was an
auspicious development, given previous judicial pronouncements to the effect
that the "violation of the person" and "the defilement," which were "inevitable
features" of stranger rape, were "not always present to the same degree when
the offender and the victim had previously had a long-standing sexual
relationship" (*R vs Berry* [1988] 10 Cr App R (S) 13). Unfortunately, however,
the court still elevated the fear caused by stranger rape, due to the "unknown
quantity" of the attacker, which may lead the victim to wonder: "[i]s he a
murderer as well as a rapist?" (*R v Millberry* [2003] 2 All ER 939, 944).

The court, however, failed to recognize the heightened fear suffered by an IPSV victim. Fear may well permeate her life, and repeat victimization is highly probable. In addition, in many cases partner rape is linked to the onset of pregnancy, thus causing additional apprehension, and a woman is also likely to suffer physical, and potentially fatal, violence (Rumney, 2003). The court also speculated that partner rape may be subject to unique forms of mitigation, due to "the ongoing nature of the relationship between the offender and the victim" (*R v Millberry* [2003] 2 All ER 939, 947) and in a case of relationship breakdown "an offender may be subject to an unusual degree of provocation or stress" (Rumney, 2003, p. 874). As discussed further below, the new 2014 Guideline may go some way to ameliorate these issues.

Not all judges regard relationship or prior relationship as a mitigating variable. Indeed, some decisions in England and Wales and in Australia have stressed both the specific trauma of a woman being raped by an estranged partner and that the parameters of aggravation should be defined the same in marital rape as in other types of sexual assault (Carline & Easteal, 2014). In quite an early Australian case, Slicer held that prior sexual relationship was not a mitigating factor, nor was the fact that marital rape had only recently been made a crime (*R v S (No 2)* [1991] Tas R 273, 280). More recently, in an Australian case of partner rape in which a man inserted a wine bottle into his partner's vagina, the appellate court stated that "[t]he fact that the complainant and the appellant were in an existing sexual relationship cannot mitigate the offence in this case" (*Gillies v DPP (NSW)* [2008] NSWCCA 339).

### Recommendation: Establish specific (or improved) sentencing legislation or guidelines

In addition to legislative amendment, establishing rape-specific sentencing guidelines in jurisdictions currently without them or improving existing ones could reduce the potential for biases or ignorance in the construction of relative harm, and of victim and perpetrator blameworthiness. In Australia, for instance, while legislative provisions such as s 21A of the *Crimes (Sentencing Procedure) Act 1999* (NSW) may guide the exercise of judicial discretion, there are no specific guidelines in relation to IPSV or indications as to the relative importance of the multiple factors to be considered. This sits in contrast with the approach adopted in England and Wales which, after a consultation process, has recently instituted a new Definitive Guideline (Sentencing Council, 2013a).

Significantly, from the inception of the consultation process (Sentencing Council, 2012), the rarity of stranger rape was acknowledged. Thus, the resulting guidance aims to encompass factors that pertain to situations where the victim knows their attacker. The Guideline further states that there is an "inherently serious" baseline of both harm and culpability in rape cases, which can only be increased (and never decreased) by the presence of other factors.

Subsequently, three categories of harm are developed, delineated according to the presence of additional factors, including severe psychological harm and threats of violence (among others). Upon determining the appropriate sentencing category, the judge will then consider the aggravating and mitigating factors. With respect to the former, this encompasses factors drawn from the domestic violence sentencing guideline, for example, compelling a victim to leave their home and the exploitation of child contact arrangements to commit an offense (Sentencing Council, 2013b: 11).

Thus, the 2014 Guideline is based upon a broader conceptualization of rape, and could be a useful template for other jurisdictions. Improvements, however, could be made. Concerns have been expressed regarding: (a) the identification of three categories of harm, as this suggests a hierarchy of rape; (b) the reduction of the minimum starting point from five to four years; and (c) the continued inclusion of remorse and good character as mitigating factors (Sentencing Council, 2013a). Furthermore, breach of trust in a partner rape should operate as an exacerbating factor. Trust should be held to encompass the reality that relationship rape can have a further-reaching and longer-lasting trauma than rape by other perpetrators.

In addition to sentencing guidelines, judges do need to be better equipped to understand the reality of rape. This can be achieved in a number of ways. Further training of court personnel is needed. Targeted training may work the best. One way of such targeting could be via "specialisation in court lists and for the creation of specialist sexual offences courts" (Heenan 2004b, para 34). Additionally, expert reports by people working in the area of violence against women and/or victim impact statements should be used routinely to facilitate an understanding of the reality of domestic violence and the particular traumas of IPSV.

## Last thoughts

The legal gatekeepers and legal provisions function within a larger social context. At the societal level, there appears to be an unconscious gendered filtering of "reality," which can militate against successful implementation of legal remedies. The existence of unwritten social subtexts is evident when we look at how IPSV is treated by the courts. Legal gatekeepers' educational and occupational subcultures often act to reinforce gender-biased beliefs and misunderstandings about violence. As a consequence, in civil and criminal remedies, police, prosecutors, magistrates, and judges may invoke stereotypes in applying the law.

The State's legal response to violence against women does need more work. However, reforms to the law should aim to empower survivors/victims and be supported by wider public messages about the reality of violence against women. We must all recognize – and that includes lawmakers and people in the community – that laws do not exist and operate in a vacuum.

# References

Australian Law Reform Commission. (2010). *Family violence – a national legal response*, report No. 114. Sydney, Australia: Author.

Basile, K. (2002). Attitudes toward wife rape: Effects of social background and victim status. *Violence and Victims, 17*(3), 341–354.

Boyle C., & MacCrimmon, M. (1998). The constitutionality of Bill C-49: Analyzing sexual assault law as if equality really mattered. *Criminal Law Quarterly, 41*(2), 198–237.

Carline, A., & Easteal P. (2014). *Shades of grey: Domestic and sexual violence against women, law reform and society*. London, UK: Routledge.

Easteal, P. (2001). *Less than equal: Women and the Australian legal system*. Sydney, Australia: Butterworths.

Easteal, P., & Gani, M. (2005). Sexual assault by male partners: A study of sentencing factors. *Southern Cross University Law Review, 9*, 39–72.

Easteal P., & McOrmond-Plummer, L. (2006). *Real rape, real pain*. Melbourne, Australia: Hybrid Press.

Edwards, K., Turchik, J., Dardis, C., Reynolds, N., & Gidycz, C. (2011). Rape myths: History, individual and institutional-level presence, and implications for change. *Sex Roles, 65*(11–12), 761–773.

Ellison, L. (2010). Commentary on R v A (No 2). In R. Hunter, C. McGlynn, & E. Rackley (Eds.), *Feminist judgments: From theory to practice* (pp. 206–210). Oxford, UK: Hart Publishing.

Ferro, C., Cermele, J., & Saltzman, A. (2008). Current perceptions of marital rape: Some good and some not-so-good news. *Journal of Interpersonal Violence, 23*(6), 764–779.

Finkelhor, D., & Yllo, K. (1985). *License to rape: Sexual abuse of wives*. New York, NY: Holt, Rinehart & Winston.

Firth, G. (2006). The rape trial and sexual history evidence – R v A and the (un)worthy complainant, *Northern Ireland Legal Quarterly, 53*(3), 442–464.

Heenan, M. (2004a). Just "keeping the peace": A reluctance to respond to male partner sexual violence. *Australian Centre for the Study of Sexual Assault Issues, 1*.

Heenan, M. (2004b) Sexual offences law and procedure, *Aware*: Australian Centre for the Study of Sexual Assault Newsletter, *5*, 8.

Hoyano, L. (2013). Case comment. R v A: Perverting the course of justice. *Criminal Law Review, 3*, 240–246.

Lazar, R. (2010). Negotiating sex: The legal construct of consent in cases of wife rape in Ontario, Canada. *Canadian Journal of Women and Law, 22*, 329–363.

Lea, S., Lanvers, U., & Shaw, S. (2003). Attrition in rape cases: Developing a profile and identifying relevant factors. *British Journal of Criminology, 43*(3), 583–599.

Long, J. (2007). Introducing expert testimony to explain victim behavior in sexual and domestic violence prosecutions. Alexandria, VA: National District Attorneys Association. Retrieved from: www.ndaa.org/pdf/pub_introducing_expert_testimony.pdf.

McGlynn, C. (2010). R v A (No 2) judgment. In R. Hunter, C. McGlynn, & E. Rackley (Eds.), *Feminist judgments: From theory to practice* (pp. 211–227). Oxford, UK: Hart Publishing.

Mahoney, P., & Williams, L. (1998). Sexual assault in marriage: Prevalence, consequences, and treatment of wife rape. In J.L. Jasinski and L.M. Williams (Eds.), *Partner violence: A comprehensive review of 20 years of research* (113–163). Thousand Oaks, CA: Sage.

Rumney, P. (2003). Progress at a price: The construction of non-stranger rape in the *Millberry* sentencing guidelines. *Modern Law Review, 66*(6), 870–884.

Sack, E.J. (2009). Is domestic violence a crime?: Intimate partner rape as allegory. *St John's Journal of Legal Commentary*, *24*(3), 535–566.

Schuller, R.A., & Hastings, P.A. (2002). Complainant sexual history evidence: Its impact on mock jurors' decisions. *Psychology of Women Quarterly*, *26*(3), 252–261.

Schuller, R.A., & Klippenstine, M.A. (2004). The impact of complainant sexual history evidence on jurors' decisions: Consideration from a psychological perspective. *Psychology, Public Policy, and Law*, *10*(3), 321–342.

Sentencing Council (2012). *Sexual Offences Guideline Consultation*. London, UK: Author.

Sentencing Council (2013a). *Research to support the development of a revised sexual offences sentencing guideline*. London, UK: Author.

Sentencing Council (2013b). *Sexual offences: Definitive guideline*. London, UK: Author.

Tadros, V. (2006). Rape without consent. *Oxford Journal of Legal Studies*, *26*(3), 515–543.

# Chapter 15

# Intimate partner sexual violence and family law

*Angela Lynch, Janet Loughman, and "Eleanor"*
*Commentary by Thomas P. Alongi*

## Introduction

Intimate partner sexual violence (IPSV), as a manifestation of family violence, is relevant within the family laws that determine parenting outcomes for children in Australia and in some U.S. states after separation.

In Australia, the paramount consideration under the *Family Law Act 1975* is the best interests of the child. In determining a child's best interests, protecting a child from physical or psychological harm from being subjected to (or exposed to) abuse, neglect, or family violence is a primary consideration of the family courts, and one that should be prioritized over the benefit to the child of having an ongoing relationship with each of their parents. Family violence, and the existence and nature of any family violence protection orders, are also relevant considerations in determining a child's best interests. A sexual assault or other sexually abusive behavior is specifically included in the examples of behavior that may constitute family violence. However, despite the legislative relevance and serious impacts of IPSV on victims/survivors and consequently their children, IPSV is rarely if ever argued – or rarely if ever argued well – in family law. This might be for a variety of reasons, including:

- Professionals within the family law system may not ask women about their experience of IPSV as they do not understand its relevance to risk.
- Women themselves have not identified their experience as IPSV.
- Women may not want to reveal their IPSV experience to lawyers and other professionals because of a lack of trust, concern that it might expose them to public scrutiny, and worry about being judged harshly.
- And raising the issue may also subject them to being cross-examined about the IPSV, which they may want to avoid.

In addition, the judiciary, lawyers, and other professionals are generally not well trained on IPSV and its impacts on adults and/or children; they may lack training on trauma more generally.

The Australian community has only just begun to have a more public conversation about the rates and impact of family violence on survivors/victims and their children. The public debate has not shifted at this stage to a more nuanced or sophisticated level, to include IPSV. IPSV, as an aspect of family violence, remains hidden from the wider public discourse. It is therefore not surprising that it also remains hidden, at worst ignored or at least minimized from legal argument and judicial outcomes in family law.

In 2011, Women's Legal Services Australia (WLSA) was approached by "Eleanor," a victim of IPSV and family violence, about her family law experience. A key role of WLSA is advocacy and law reform. This chapter includes Eleanor's experiences and builds on previous work of WLSA, in particular the work of Pasanna Mutha. We also report on our findings from a 2015 WLSA survey of 330 survivors of domestic and family violence to gather evidence about the extent and impact of the experience of being directly cross-examined in family law courts (Loughman, 2016; Lynch, 2015). Note that both in reporting survey responses and in Eleanor's story, details have been slightly altered for the purposes of deidentification and compliance with s. 121 of the *Family Law Act 1975*.

High levels of violence were reported in the survey, including 64% of women reporting sexual violence. We are unsure whether the IPSV was disclosed to the court. What we know, however, is if these survey respondents who identified they had experienced sexual violence had reported this to the police and criminal proceedings were commenced, their perpetrator would not have been allowed to cross-examine them directly in the state criminal courts. Victims of IPSV receive no similar protection in family law. The prevalence of IPSV among respondents highlights the importance of current inconsistent approaches within Australian court systems. Family law is out of step in protecting victims of IPSV and family violence.

## Co-parenting and IPSV

In Eleanor's parenting case, the judgment from the Federal Magistrates Court (now known as the Federal Circuit Court) ordered equal shared parental responsibility of the children between Eleanor and her former husband. This order obligated Eleanor to negotiate with her former husband to try to reach agreement about any issues that had a long-term impact on the children (such as medical issues, religion, counseling for the children, and schooling). Eleanor asked a very valid question, "How do I co-parent with my rapist?" It is also clear from Eleanor's own words that as a survivor of IPSV, she confronted the following challenges:

- what is colloquially known as the "future focus of family law proceedings" – that is, a requirement or attitude of professionals and the broader system

that directs parties within the system to look to the future rather than "rehashing past wrongs" that can result in allegations of violence and abuse not being raised and survivors' experiences being silenced;
* the lack of expertise and knowledge about IPSV by professionals within the system;
* the ongoing and powerful myth in family law that a perpetrator of IPSV and family violence can be a good father despite being a bad husband.

These attitudes are evidenced in the words of Eleanor's own barrister when he told her, "They (the court) don't care that he raped you, it's about his relationship with his children and the sooner you get used to that the better."

## IPSV and cross-examination in other (non-family) courts

In each Australian State and Territory there are legal protections in many civil and criminal proceedings to prevent unrepresented litigants from cross-examining former partners where there is a history of violence, including sexual violence. These protections recognize the traumatic impact of cross-examination on victims of violence by their own perpetrators. There are no equivalent protections in family law.

In state jurisdictions such as Victoria, Tasmania, Western Australia, and South Australia, an unrepresented accused person in a civil law domestic violence protection order matter cannot directly cross-examine the protected person who is the subject of proceedings. Section 70 of the *Family Violence Protection Act 2008* (Vic) applies in Victoria. It provides an exception where the protected person is an adult, consents, and the court decides it would not have a harmful impact upon the protected person. The protection also extends to children, family members of the protected person, and anyone else declared to be a protected person. Section 8A(1) of the *Evidence (Children and Special Witnesses) Act 2001* (Tas) applies in Tasmania. Section 3 provides that the protection applies to anyone giving evidence in respect of family violence as defined by the *Family Violence Act 2004* (Tas), as well as a number of those who are alleged victims of certain crimes enumerated in the Criminal Code, the *Sex Industry Offenses Act 2005* (Tas) the *Police Offenses Act 1935* (Tas) and the *Classification (Publications, Films and Computer Games) Enforcement Act 1995* (Tas). Section 44C of the *Restraining Orders Act 1997* (WA) applies. The protection extends to any person who is in a family and domestic relationship or an imagined relationship with the defendant (the "imagined relationship" refers to a stalker who believes there is an intimate relationship that does not exist (Creek, n.d.)). Section 44C(2) provides that the section does not apply if the witness requests that it should not, or if the court considers that it should not apply in the interests of justice. Section 29(4)(a) of the *Intervention Orders (Prevention of Abuse) Act 2009* (SA) provides that the protection extends to a person against whom it is alleged the defendant has committed an act of abuse, or a child against whom abuse is alleged or who might be subject to abuse.

In South Australia, Western Australia, the Northern Territory, and Victoria, under *Intervention Orders (Prevention of Abuse) Act 2009* (SA), s 29(4)(b); *Restraining Orders Act 1997* (WA), s 44C(1)(d); *Domestic and Family Violence Act 2007* (NT), s 114(3); *Family Violence Protection Act 2008* (Vic), s 71, a person is appointed by the court to carry out the cross-examination. In Victoria, this person is appointed by Legal Aid, while in the other jurisdictions the respondent must pose his or her questions to the court or a person appointed by the court, who must repeat those questions accurately to the complainant.

### Vulnerable witnesses in sexual offense trials

In all Australian state jurisdictions an unrepresented accused person in a sexual offense proceeding cannot directly cross-examine the complainant. These include:

- *Criminal Procedure Act 1986* (NSW), s 294A, where the protection applies to the complainant of a prescribed sexual offense;
- *Evidence (Miscellaneous Provisions) Act 1991* (ACT), s 38D(4), where the protection applies to a complainant or similar act witness in a prescribed sexual offense;
- *Criminal Procedure Act 2009* (Vic), s 365, where the protection applies to a complainant, family member of the complainant, family member of the accused, or anyone else declared to be a protected witness in a charge relating to a sexual offense;
- *Evidence (Children and Special Witnesses) Act 2001* (Tas), s 8A(1), where the protection applies to anyone giving evidence in respect of family violence as defined by the *Family Violence Act 2004* (Tas), as well those who are alleged victims of certain crimes enumerated in the Criminal Code;
- the *Sex Industry Offenses Act 2005* (Tas), the *Police Offenses Act 1935* (Tas), and the *Classification (Publications, Films and Computer Games) Enforcement Act 1995* (Tas);
- *Evidence Act 1929* (SA), s 13B, where the protection applies to the alleged victim of any serious offense against the person, and offenses of contravening or failing to comply with an intervention or restraining order;
- *Sexual Offenses (Evidence and Procedure) Act* (NT), s 5(1)(a), where the protection relates to the complainant of a prescribed sexual offense;
- *Evidence Act 1977* (Qld), s 21N, where the protection applies to any victim of a number of prescribed special offenses under the Criminal Code, or the victim of a prescribed offense under the Criminal Code where the Court considers that they would be likely to suffer emotional trauma or be disadvantaged as a witness unless treated as a protected person;

- *Evidence Act 1906* (WA), s 106G, where the protection extends to the victim of a serious sexual offense unless they consent to the protection not applying.

In Tasmania, *Evidence (Children and Special Witnesses) Act 2001* (Tas), s 8A. and South Australia, *Evidence Act 1929* (SA), s 13B the accused must obtain legal representation or forfeit the right to cross-examination.

In all other Australian jurisdictions, a person is appointed to carry out the cross-examination. In Victoria (section 357(2) *Criminal Procedure Act 2009* (Vic) and Queensland (*Evidence Act 1977* (Qld) s 210), this person is appointed by the statutory Legal Aid body (*Evidence Act 1977* (Qld) s 219). In New South Wales (*Criminal Procedure Act 1986* (NSW) s 294A), the court must appoint the person.

### Protections for vulnerable witnesses in commonwealth criminal trials

In 2013, federal protections were introduced for adult complainants in proceedings under the *Crimes Act 1914*, relating to slavery and slavery-like conditions as well as trafficking in persons or debt bondage: *Crimes Act 1914* (Cth) s 15YG.

## What can the courts do now to prevent cross-examination by perpetrators in family law in Australia?

The *Family Law Act* contains no protection against direct cross-examination by perpetrators or any specific protections in general – for example, for witnesses with disability. As Eleanor experienced:

A week later I was back in that same courtroom for family law proceedings. I was sick to my stomach to discover on day one of the hearing that he had become a self litigant and was going to be directly cross-examining me.

I did not want retribution; I wanted to leave my perpetrator, heal, and have a good life. The system was meant to be there to protect me in doing this. So many times I had heard people say "She should just leave," but when you do, it's like jumping out of a plane and the system is meant to be your parachute but each time you pull on the cord it just won't open.

He had effectively exhausted me emotionally, physically, and financially, and had used every system at his disposal to inflict as much trauma and pressure on me that he could.

That day I stood on the stand and the federal court allowed him to directly cross-examine me was a massive slap in the face. How could they give my rapist his power back over me? He asked questions I was forced to answer; he was only meters from me . . . How could this happen when another magistrate had said that this circumstance was not appropriate or safe for me?

It is this system flaw that I was able to identify as a major flaw and obstacle in my recovery from trauma. Having your rapist stand only meters from you asking intimate and personal questions about your relationships, your parenting, your social media accounts, every aspect of your personal life is invasive, disempowering, and cruel. This person does not deserve the right to directly cross-examine their victim.

Judges in family law proceedings can use the *Family Law Act* provisions in Part VII Division 12A, including the principles outlined in section 69ZN, to ensure that the proceedings are conducted in a way that will safeguard the parties. These can usefully be applied to allow parties to use a safe room at court; to give evidence by video link; and for an Independent Children's Lawyer (ICL) to cross-examine first, prior to an unrepresented litigant, when an ICL is present in a case. The judicial officer can intervene to restrict inappropriate questions to the extent that he or she feels fairness allows and an appeal will not result (if inappropriate questions can be identified, since this can be difficult in intimate partner violence and arguably even more so in IPSV).

Although these measures assist, they do not adequately remedy the injustice that flows and that other proceedings such as sexual assault trials have some time ago accommodated. There are also real questions that must be asked about the judiciary's ability to identify trauma or trauma responses in witnesses and appropriately intervene.

Some of our survey respondents commented on the failure of the court to either recognize their trauma and/or to take adequate steps to intervene and protect them.

> I felt frozen, on the outside looking normal, on the inside like I was bound and gagged. His tactics and lies were treated as truth; he had direct contact to all the barristers and lawyers. I was silenced. I could not look at him.

> Terrifying. I could not look at him. The judge later said in his submission that I hated the man cause I couldn't look at him. The man terrorized me for years and to this day is still making me paranoid that he will carry out his death threat.

Many described a feeling that they were fighting not only their own perpetrator, but also the legal system and clearly identified that the "system" was complicit in their abuse, by allowing their perpetrator direct access to them while giving evidence:

I felt he had the privilege to continue his intimidation and threats yet in a confined legal space. It defeats the purpose of having a safety room at court – my support person and I sit there to avoid seeing him yet we are "thrown to the wolves" when we enter the courtroom. It made me feel all the feelings over again, it made me sick to the core.

Absolutely broken, angry at our justice system, scared.

Horrible, it was just horrible. It felt like he was given a stick to beat me whilst everybody watched.

## Impact of cross-examination by abusers

Cross-examination by an alleged abuser has a devastating impact when experienced, and can also lead to some women choosing to settle their family law matter on less than satisfactory terms to avoid being cross-examined by – or having to cross-examine – a violent perpetrator of IPSV or other family violence. For example, the survey found that 39% of matters were settled before judgment, and 45% of these respondents said that the prospective fear of personal cross-examination by their abuser was a factor in their decision to settle; 71% identified it as a significant issue. This adds weight to the concern that victims of IPSV and more broadly victims of family violence may be settling their family law matters because they are frightened and intimidated by the prospect of direct cross-examination and arguably in circumstances that may not be in the best interests of children.

### Impact on the quality of the evidence

The experience of being cross-examined by a perpetrator can compromise the quality of evidence given to the court, which can affect the court's ability to make safe and effective orders, and can allow the perpetrator to use court proceedings to exercise control and dominance over the victim. Some respondents reported minimizing the violence and essentially changing their evidence out of fear of their perpetrator:

I knew he was going to cross-examine me, and so I purposefully did not bring up the abuse I endured. I tried, but I couldn't. I was too scared of him cross-examining me on that issue. He exerted so much control over me that I was too scared to raise it at all.

I played down everything; I still was controlled by him due to years of conditioning. Knowing the consequences if I had answered truthfully. The tone, the way he asked questions. There was so much more to everything than what everyone heard. He walked out winning again. I had the kids but on his terms.

To make the best decisions the court requires the best evidence. It is questionable whether allowing a perpetrator direct access to their victim in the witness box results in the best outcome for the child (the subject of the dispute), the victim or the family. These survey results are extremely concerning and provide evidence that allowing an alleged perpetrator to directly cross-examine their victim affects not only the quality and type of evidence that is presented to the court, but may well fundamentally compromise the efficacy of the entire trial process.

### Retrauma

A total of 144 respondents made comments about the effect that the cross-examination had on them. Three respondents spoke about being suicidal, having their medication increased, and having difficulty in day-to-day functioning after the personal cross-examination. Many spoke about having their posttraumatic stress disorder symptoms triggered. One respondent reported needing medication to get into the courtroom and having a nervous breakdown as a result of the experience. Many felt physically ill at the prospect of the cross-examination, during the process, and afterwards. Another described having her disability exacerbated.

Eleanor's words detail the devastating impact on her psychological health of being personally cross-examined by her former husband, her own abuser, as he was representing himself without a lawyer in their family law trial:

> As I stood there, the flashbacks of him raping me, of violently kicking me with his steel-capped boots, him screaming at me that he could not stand the smell of me . . . was all I could hear. His questions to all around would have seemed standard or at the very most mildly intrusive but for me standing there being forced to answer him each time he spoke to me was soul-wrenching.
>
> I ran from the room, hyperventilating, consumed in trauma . . . I could not breathe, I could not think, I could only feel him all around me. His voice in my head, his hands around my throat, his complete hatred of me . . . . I was saturated in him . . . again . . . and the judge allowed it to happen.
>
> There are currently clauses that allow a judge to use their discretion as to whether this cross-examination occurs. This is not sufficient . . . real law changes need to happen.
>
> This man did so many cruel and hurtful things to me – criminal events. . . . We need the law to firmly state that this should never happen.
>
> I wanted to end my life that day. . . . I wanted the torture to end. I could see no future ahead of me that did not have my perpetrator pulling all the strings.
>
> I had to split that person . . . I had to try and see him through an imaginary lens where I could pretend he was a good father where I could

trust my children in his care . . . because the courts decided that was what would happen . . . I had to accept this despite the injustice. I accepted the shared parenting agreement and the sentence of co-parenting I was given till my daughter turns 18. It had never been about the children . . . it was about using the system to be able to wield his power over me. And the system gave it to him.

I survived my abuser and the system he dragged me through . . . but I recognize so many others do not! They do not have either the support from family and friends, the financial means, or the luxury of a Master's degree to help navigate themselves through such a tortuous system.

## Cross-examination by lawyers

Although the survey sought to elicit information specifically about survivors' experiences of being directly cross-examined by their own abuser, two respondents identified concerns about the conduct of cross-examination more broadly in circumstances of IPSV and/or family violence, even when conducted by a lawyer.

A lawyer may have been more successful at being brutal toward me – many lawyers are as verbally brutal as their clients.

My ex-partner's lawyer brutalized me in open court about a sexual assault that had occurred.

## Advocating for change: The voice of Eleanor

I am only one victim of the system. There are thousands of victims just like me who are too afraid or damaged to speak out.

I believe as a community we can do better. Most states amended their laws in 2008 in civil cases so that alleged perpetrators were not given the opportunity to cross-examine their victims. The federal system is lagging.

I began writing letters to all who would listen. I have corresponded and met with federal leaders and representatives. I have received sympathy and empathy for the predicament I and other women have been placed in, but what I haven't received is real action by the federal government on this issue. It seems simple to me no person, male or female, should be cross-examined by the person who raped and beat them. When I had no joy from local members and from the attorney general I began to turn to the media.

My letters and emails came before the likes of Angela Lynch and Pasanna Mutha who have taken on this issue in the media and at high levels in government. These women have been relentless and beside me in addressing this flaw. Working with WLSA has helped me to politicize this issue and keep it in the forefront of discussion in a variety of forums. Angela and Pasanna were able to provide the legal knowledge of how this change could occur. I was an example of the "Why."

I have had to use a false name due to restraints of the family law system . . . I chose Eleanor. In the media the voice of Eleanor has been loud and has been heard. The headline is catchy I guess and a shock for many. How can our community allow a victim of violence to be cross-examined by their abuser? It sounds dreadful, doesn't it? But not dreadful enough for the government to amend its laws and use other avenues to stop this event from happening to victims on a daily basis.

The voice of Eleanor has enabled me to speak on the behalf of those who have no voice, who are unable to fight for change as they are fighting too hard to survive each day. It has enabled me to talk to important people like yourselves who each day deal with victims of violence who are restricted and challenged in a system that should be supporting them and helping them to recover and progress as a protective parent.

This is not about stopping parents from seeing their children . . . it is not about stopping them from having the right to cross-examine . . . it is about protecting victims of violence in order to assist them to recover and heal from their trauma and be the best parents they can be for their children.

## Box 15.1 Cross-examination by perpetrators in family law in the United States

*Commentary by Thomas P. Alongi*

A framework of laws already exists that would regularly vindicate a survivor's (and her child's) interest in safety and a life of relative peace . . . if only family court participants educated themselves, swept away their subconscious biases, and vigorously met both political correctness and junk behavioral science head on. More than a new rule, we need a community willingness to transform survivors' lives using laws we already have. We do not fail because of statutory loopholes; we stumble because – in the end – we still do not understand IPV.

It is unlikely that Eleanor's proposal would muster popular support in the United States, or survive constitutional scrutiny even if it did – at least to the extent it substantially curtailed cross-examination. Both Australia and America descend from a British tradition of common law, but with important differences. For example, and by way of contrast, Eleanor cites the Australian courts' ability to restrain such examinations in criminal and order of protection hearings. That luxury is largely nonexistent in the United States. The Confrontation

Clause to the Sixth Amendment assures a criminal defendant of the opportunity to confront his accuser, literally "face-to-face." This is true even if the Rules of Evidence would otherwise permit the government to use an absent survivor's statements because of a hearsay exception long accepted under common law. Ironically, this constitutional guarantee exists – in part – precisely *because* such personal confrontations ensure the trier of fact's ability to observe demeanor, nervousness, expressions, and other body language of the witness (see *United States v. Hamilton,* 107 F.3d 499, 503 (7th Cir. 1997).

This is an important consideration. Our legal system cannot assume the truth of an allegation of criminal behavior, no matter the arena; otherwise, we effectively presume guilt absent proof of innocence. No self-respecting constitutional republic could ever tolerate such a guiding principle, as it would necessarily apply in every context – not just for the sake of IPSV survivors. Therefore, the ideal solution to this challenging and complex problem would provide a forum that (a) imparts the severity of such proceedings and dire consequences of perjured testimony on everyone, yet (b) avoids the needless psychological paralysis of a truthful survivor.

The American justice system has commended cross-examination as "the greatest legal engine ever invented for the discovery of the truth" (*California v. Green,* 399 U.S. 149, 158 (1970), *citing* 5 Wigmore § 1367). As an attorney who regularly represents IPV survivors in family court, I can scarcely complain. The ability to force an evasive, dishonest batterer to answer all those uncomfortable "yes or no" questions about his violence, manipulations, and psychological cruelty behind closed doors is not a litigation tool that I (or any other victim's advocate) should lightly dilute or surrender.

Certainly, there is recent movement afoot to ease the process for a sexual assault survivor to give testimony in administrative proceedings, such as a university board hearing aimed at the possible suspension or expulsion of a fellow student. Such procedures include "conduit examination," where the accused student must funnel questions to the hearing panel, which then decides if the question has merit and (if so) voices the question to the alleged victim. But even previous administrative processes came under fire for their claimed lack of fidelity to due process. See, e.g., *Winnick v. Manning,* 460 F.2d 545 (2nd Cir. 1972) and *Blanton v. State University of New York,* 489 F.2d 377 (2nd Cir. 1973); see also Triplett, "Sexual Assault on College Campuses: Seeking the Appropriate Balance Between Due Process and Victim Protection," 62 DUKE L. J. 487, 512–17 (2012) (identifying heightened due process worries, and suggesting unique procedures, for school disciplinary hearings adjudicating allegations of peer sexual assault).

And American courts have drawn a firm line between administrative hearings and civil courtrooms, including family law proceedings. Indeed, one could hardly expect a looser approach regarding families, since the ability to raise a child is regarded as a fundamental constitutional right. See *Stanley v. Illinois*, 405 U.S. 645, 651 (1972) (recognizing unwed father's right to evidentiary fitness hearing before children could be removed from his care as "dependent"); *Santosky v. Kramer*, 455 U.S. 745, 753 (1982) (imposing "clear and convincing" standard for parental severance cases as a matter of due process).

We can explore trial methods that promote a search for the truth and require an alleged victim's personal participation, while still blunting an offender's zeal for face-to-face trauma. But we cannot dispense wholesale with cross-examination by an unrepresented abuser. Yet with twenty-first-century Internet tools now at our disposal, solutions such as remote testimony via Skype, iMeet, or Facetime appear well within our reach, especially as courtrooms continue to modernize. And even today, pure telephonic testimony is permitted on a showing of need. See ARIZ. R. FAM. L. P. 8.

We must do more than modify rules of witness examination. Even where a victim secures permission to log into the courtroom via broadband Internet access and voices her tribulation beyond all hope, we have not assured anyone the court will understand IPV dynamics sufficiently to apply those principles in a decision that rescues vulnerable children. The education process must continue relentlessly. Family court stakeholders must come to understand batterer and survivor behaviors both pre- and post-separation. They must appreciate the inescapable trilemma encountered by every IPV survivor with children: (1) remain in the home, and endure further violence along with risk of intervention by a child welfare agency for her "failure to protect," (2) flee with the children, and invite a criminal charge of kidnapping, or (3) flee without the children, and accept near-universal condemnation as an unfit mother who has "abandoned" her own offspring.

## Conclusion

The responses to the Australian survey confirm significant issues and barriers to survivors of IPSV accessing justice from the family law system. We need to support survivors throughout their legal journey after separation, including through the family law system. They require access to adequate legal aid, as the existence of a lawyer may provide some protection. As a matter of urgency, legislative protections in family law should be introduced to stop direct cross-examination of survivors by their alleged abusers. In addition, the *Family Law*

*Act* needs to be amended to remove its emphasis on shared parenting to deincentivize against perpetrators using legal processes for the purposes of exerting ongoing control and intimidation. The family law system as a whole needs to undergo significant redesign to make it more responsive to IPSV, trauma, and family violence. Consideration should also be given to the development of guidelines or protocols that outline acceptable standards of cross-examination, even when conducted by a lawyer, given the levels of trauma experienced by users within the family law system.

## References

Creek, S. (n.d.). Court ordered boundaries in shifting relationships. Retrieved from: myFamilyLaw website: http://myfamilylaw.net.au/court-ordered-boundaries-shifting-relationships.

Loughman, J. (2016, February). Protecting vulnerable witnesses in family law. *Law Society of NSW Journal*, 26–27.

Lynch, A. (2015, December). Thrown to the wolves: Survey responses of female victims/ survivors of domestic/family violence, the family courts and cross examination. Presentation at Stop Domestic Violence: Connecting the Dots Conference, Canberra, Australia.

# Chapter 16

# When intimate partner sexual violence intersects with faith traditions and practices

*Marie M. Fortune*

## The fact of faith

In the 1990s, an article appeared describing a court case where a convicted wife abuser attempted to use the First Amendment of the U.S. Constitution as his defense against a charge of marital rape of his wife. He argued that the Roman Catholic Church had taught him that he had the right to have sex with his wife at any time because their marriage vows signaled her permanent consent to sexual activity. He sought to justify breaking into her locked room, slapping her, and ripping her clothing as legitimate foreplay justified by the Church and protected by the First Amendment free exercise of religious beliefs (Abrahamson, 1996). The court was not impressed and he was convicted.

The media immediately went to the local archdiocese asking for comment. The archdiocesan representative clarified that no, this was not the Church's teaching and that husbands and wives should treat each other with mutual respect. But the representative was silent and did not name this woman's experience as "marital rape" or "domestic violence" or a "sin." The Church had the opportunity to step up and stand with the victim/survivor as well as call the perpetrator to account, but it did not.

In researching this chapter, I have been amazed at the paucity of discussion of "marital rape" in most religious commentaries on marriage and sexuality. The assumption of a husband's sexual access to his wife is so deeply ingrained in religious and cultural traditions that it generally does not even appear as a topic for discussion. If it does appear, it simply reinforces the assumption as we see in this nineteenth-century directive:

> No woman then should ever marry without a full knowledge of her duties to her husband, particularly in the sexual respect; for without granting this privilege to her husband in full and free accord, there *cannot* be maintained a happy married life ... Quite too many cases have come under my observation where the marriage vow has never been consummated or, if consummated at all, in a very begrudging manner, owing to the

*insubordination* [italics mine] of the wife . . . This is not only wrong, but it is a most unpardonable vice.

(Guernsey, 1882, pp. 94–95)

Needless to say, the words "consent" or "mutuality" do not appear in this text.

This assumption of a husband's sexual access to a wife supports the erroneous belief in many faith communities that there is no such thing as "marital rape" or sexual violence in intimate relationships. This is still evident in the adage, "You can't rape your wife." Under these circumstances, the dynamics of a heterosexual, intimate relationship continue to be assumed to be male sexual access to a woman partner with or without consent. This assumption flourishes in an ideological context of female submission and male entitlement which Adrienne Rich describes as "husband right":"

. . . one specific form of the rights men are presumed to enjoy simply because of their gender: the "right" to the priority of male over female needs, to sexual and emotional services from women, to women's undivided attention in any or all situations . . .

(Rich, 1979, pp. 219–220)

Sadly, "husband right" describes the cultural norms and expectations promulgated by some in our various religious traditions. It is the dominant–submissive model of intimacy that sets the stage for intimate partner sexual violence (IPSV).

## The historical view

We finally begin to see the discussion of IPSV and religion starting in the late 1970s in *Conjugal crime* (Davidson, 1978) and the 1980s with *Sexual violence: The unmentionable sin* (Fortune, 1983) in my discussion of "marital rape" in the context of consent (p. 105) and in *Keeping the faith: Guidance for Christian women facing abuse* (Fortune, 1987, pp. 16–17). In *Abuse and religion: When praying isn't enough* (Horton & Williamson, 1988), Kersti Yllo and Donna LeClerc address religion in their article "Marital rape." Horton and Williamson's volume was one of the first anthologies to address religion and intimate partner violence (IPV). Also Pamela Cooper-White offers an explicit discussion of marital rape in *The cry of Tamar: Violence against women and the Church's response*, 1995. Additionally, in 1995, in *Love does no harm*, I offer an extensive discussion of the moral norm of consent in sexually intimate relationships.

Rather than directly addressing the issue of IPSV, religions approach the topic through two different lenses: sexual violence in general (such as prohibitions against rape) and definitions of marriage and what is expected of intimate partners. This is important when considering how religions address both larger categories. The religious context theoretically promotes an ethical framework in matters of marriage (assumed to be heterosexual) and sexual behavior.

Historically, religious teachings have sought to regulate sexual behavior by relegating it to "marriage only" but have rarely addressed the qualitative nature of this intimate relationship.

## Two aspects of IPSV and faith

This chapter addresses, then, not only intimate partner violence which includes sexual violence, but also intimate relationships absent the pattern of coercive control (enforced by physical threat and violence) but with the assumption of sexual access by the male to the female in the context of entitlement. IPSV can occur in either circumstance. The difference between rape, forced sex, coercive sex, or nonconsensual sex is a matter of degree, not substance. A similar distinction is made by Yllo and LeClerc: "battering rapes," "force only rapes," and "other," which includes coercive sex related to pornography (Yllo & LeClerc, 1988, pp. 54–55). The substantive ethical and pastoral issue here is the absence of authentic consent between adult intimate partners, whether because of explicit violence or an implicit, unquestioned assumption of sexual access founded in religious and/or cultural gender expectations.

The assumption is that male dominance and female submission are the natural order of things; this extends to an intimate sexual relationship in some religious traditions and contemporary expressions. In this, historically, religion has been in service to patriarchal values, customs, and norms.

Religious teaching and doctrine may manifest as either a roadblock to a healthy, consensual intimate relationship or a resource to the same. This means that distorted, misused religious texts and teachings can easily be used to excuse or justify bad, abusive behavior in an intimate relationship. Likewise, they can be used to confront and correct bad behavior and establish norms for healthy relationships.

## Islam, Judaism, and Christianity

The remainder of this chapter will focus on the issues of consent in intimate relationships in the three primary Western Abrahamic traditions of Judaism, Islam, and Christianity, with an emphasis on teaching, sacred texts, and doctrines; how these elements of religious traditions have been misused to justify and to ignore IPSV; and the possible alternatives to address and confront IPSV within the traditions themselves.

### Islam

Contrary to some public stereotypes of Muslim marriage relationships, the Qur'an and the Sunnah are very explicit about the mutuality of marriage and the protection of women's rights not to be exploited by an abusive husband.

Unfortunately, as in other faith traditions, local customs have too often reflected patriarchal values contrary to these fundamental teachings.

Salma Abugideiri and Imam Mohamed Hag Magid have written a remarkable guide for Muslim couples preparing to marry (Abugideiri & Magid, 2014). An Islamic marriage is based on a contract between spouses: a prenuptial agreement, and the moral terms and conditions. Both spouses can specify financial arrangements, monogamy, the right to work outside the home, and other aspects of their relationship. Any violation of the contract will be grounds for an Islamic divorce.

The preparation of these contracts allows for a useful pre-marriage process which addresses many significant issues. Of course, this process is only useful if it is taken seriously by both parties. According to Abugideiri and Magid (2014), "The Islamic model of marriage is a preventive one that is designed to protect the health of the marital relationship" (p. 149).

The principles derived from the Qur'an and Sunnah are:

- "kindness" (no abuse of any kind);
- "protection of the integrity of the marriage" (fidelity and meeting each other's emotional and sexual needs);
- "mutual protection" (care for the other);
- "loyalty" (monogamy and protection of privacy);
- "intimacy" (to provide for the mutual enjoyment of each other);
- "letting each other go with kindness" (divorce if the marriage is not working).

What is most interesting about Islamic teaching about marital relationships is the emphasis on discussion of sexual intimacy and an effort to offer guidance to encourage mutuality and dialogue for a healthy intimate relationship. "The Prophet (pbuh [peace be upon him]) warned men not to approach their wives like animals, and encouraged foreplay as part of a healthy and mutually satisfying intimate relationship" (Abugideiri & Magid, 2014, p. 165). Also "the Prophet (pbuh) expressed his disapproval for men who beat their wives during the day, then wanted to be intimate with them at night" (p. 166). In speaking of intimacy, Abugideiri and Magid state:

> The abuse we see in some relationships, like marital rape, reflects a misunderstanding of this right. It is not true that this right can be demanded anytime, regardless of circumstances, with no respect to the emotional state of the other person. . . . Intimacy cannot be withheld nor can it be forced.
> (pp. 151–153)

The explicit references to intimate partner sexual violence and the emphasis on teaching values of mutuality and respect are a significant contribution to this discussion from Islamic teaching.

## Judaism

Again, if we look to the sacred texts and teachings of Judaism, we generally find a sex-affirmative context. The emphasis in the discussion of marital intimacy (because all sexual activity is assumed to be within heterosexual marriage) is on the nature of consent. But, like in Islam, the discussion is often explicit and the ethical norms very clear. Mark Dratch, a modern Orthodox rabbi, in his article "I do? Consent and coercion in sexual relations," addresses rape in general and marital rape in particular (Dratch, 2014). The Torah compares rape to murder (Deut. 22:26), which clearly asserts that rape is violent assault, not sex. This clarity serves as foundational to an understanding of intimate partner sexual violence in a Jewish relationship. There remains, however, a subtext of property ownership and the woman's assault by a man other than her husband is described as an assault against the husband because his property is damaged (see the unnamed concubine in Judges 19). This creates something of a contradiction of ethical norms and a silencing of the woman's experience. However, in marriage, Dratch summarizes:

> It is forbidden for a man to force his wife to have intercourse. Even if she is not forced outright, as long as she is not amenable to intercourse, sexual relations are prohibited . . . Even if she is ambivalent about her desire, relations are forbidden.
>
> (Dratch, 2014, p. 597)

Jewish marriage assumes that husbands and wives will satisfy the sexual needs of each other. This is explicit and foundational to the marriage covenant but always with the expectation of consent. "But this obligation [of sexual availability to each other] is not absolute and does not offer unconstrained license to a husband to be with his wife whenever he wants" (Dratch, p. 604). This explicit teaching addresses "force only" or nonconsensual intimate partner sexual violence but it does not address "battering" sexual violence.

Since the 1980s, many Jewish movements in the U.S. and elsewhere have addressed domestic violence in the Jewish family. Here, they have drawn on specific teachings such as *Shalom Bayit* (peace in the home) and *Pikuach Nefesh* (to save a life or the obligation to safeguard the health and well-being of another person above all else). These are significant resources to support healthy Jewish marriage and family life.

## Christianity

The context of addressing the particulars of IPSV in Christian marriage rests on two principles which arise from questionable interpretation of sacred texts: the subordination of women to men and husbands' right of chastisement.

The most common text cited in reference to subordination is Ephesians Chapter 5 (New Revised Standard Version (NSRV)): "Wives, be subject to your husbands as you are to the Lord. For the husband is the head of the wife just as Christ is the head of the Church, the body of which he is the Savior" (vv. 22–23). But the passage goes on: "In the same way, husbands should love their wives as they do their own bodies. He who loves his wife loves himself" (v. 28). The most significant verse in this passage precedes "wives be subject to husbands": "Be subject to one another out of reverence for Christ" (v. 21). This is the foundational principle of mutuality in relationships that challenges the dominance–submission model of marriage. The passage also gives extensive instructions to husbands on proper treatment of wives including Jesus' relationship with the Church as the model of husbands' relationships to wives.

The right of chastisement appears in Church teaching in the Middle Ages. In *The rules of marriage*, a fifteenth-century marriage manual, we read:

> [in response to a wife's disobedience] . . . Scold her sharply, bully and terrify her. And if this still doesn't work . . . take up a stick and beat her soundly, for it is better to punish the body and correct the soul than to damage the soul and spare the body . . .
>
> (Davidson, 1978, p. 99)

Although this teaching was not biblically based, it was nonetheless significant and consistent with legal standards and customs in that period. Based on these two assumptions, husbands could assume that they are entitled to sexual access to wives at any time and if a wife refuses, she has challenged his authority and can be punished for it.

The specific Christian biblical text that is still often misused to address IPSV is found in 1 Corinthians Chapter 7 (NRSV): "The husband should give to his wife her conjugal rights, and likewise the wife to her husband. For the wife does not have authority over her own body, but the husband does; likewise the husband does not have authority over his own body, but the wife does" (vv. 3–4). This explicit standard for mutuality in marital intimacy could not be more clear. The expectation is that a couple's sexual relationship will be negotiated to meet both their needs with no justification of coercion or force involved.

The problem of the lack of clear discussion of marital rape or the issue of consent in Christian marriage extends late into the twentieth century. For example, in the chapter "The unity of the marital act" by John B. Gruenenfelder (1972), we find an extensive discussion of heterosexual intercourse in marriage as an ontological act of union: "To say that sexual unity is natural means primarily that it is fit, right, appropriate and proportionate to conjugal love. It is just. It is an act in which the loving being manifests itself" (Gruenenfelder, p. 108). It is an affirmation of heterosexual marital intimacy (not based on procreation) by definition deemed just with no qualifiers. But there is never any mention of consent except to say, "The fact that intercourse can be bestial and rapist does not gainsay the point" (Gruenenfelder, p. 107).

In the early twenty-first century, we find a new variation on an old theme revealing the current theological gymnastics to justify sexual coercion in Christian marriage. This commentary comes from Pastor Doug Wilson (Anne, 2012), a prominent evangelical leader:

> The final aspect of rape that should be briefly mentioned is perhaps closer to home. Because we have forgotten the biblical concepts of true authority and submission, or more accurately, have rebelled against them, we have created a climate in which caricatures of authority and submission intrude upon our lives with violence . . . . the sexual act cannot be made into an egalitarian pleasuring party. A man penetrates, conquers, plants. A woman receives, surrenders, accepts . . . True authority and true submission are therefore an erotic necessity.

Former megachurch pastor Mark Driscoll (2014) elaborates on this idea, asserting that woman was created to be a "home" for a man's penis. Again, we find no discussion of consent or mutuality as fundamental to heterosexual marital intimacy.

While faith leaders like Doug Wilson and Mark Driscoll do not represent mainstream Protestant or Catholic thought on this subject, they do represent a significant message still being preached in many churches. In addition, we find efforts to actually justify "wife abuse" using Christian theology. Bruce Ware, professor of Christian Theology at Southern Baptist Theological Seminary in Louisville, Kentucky, argues that the reason husbands abuse their wives is that women rebel against men's authority (Allen, 2008). This blaming-the-victim strategy never challenges the basic model of dominance and subordination but rather accepts it as part of the natural order. This is the way things are and should be accepted as such.

### Commonalities in the three traditions

Within our religious traditions, the sacred texts, teachings and rhetoric are there to challenge these interpretations. We find multiple resources to shape ethical and pastoral understanding of critical issues like IPSV. Custom and practice too often ignore these fundamental teachings and even attempt to reference religious sources to justify IPSV. The more disturbing result of this survey of teachings and practices of Christianity, Judaism, and Islam is the virtual absence of mention of marital rape or of the expectation of consent in marital intimacy. This silence speaks volumes.

## So what does a faith leader do?

Carol Adams begins her article, "I just raped my wife! what are you going to do about it, Pastor?" (Adams, 1993), with a story about Shirley, a victim of physical and sexual violence at the hands of her husband. She went to her pastor; he counseled her to forgive. When she literally phoned the pastor during an assault, her abuser got on the phone and taunted the pastor.

This incident illustrates the multiple challenges faced by a faith leader who learns of IPSV. First is the question of who discloses the abuse. Does the victim/survivor come seeking help and support, or does the abuser come confessing and ready to repent and seek help? It is unusual for the abuser to come confessing unless he has been confronted by a sermon or conversation that reaches his conscience and breaks through his denial that he has a problem. It is less unusual for the victim/survivor to come forward and disclose. But even here she is at great risk to disclose to a faith leader unless she has some signal that the faith leader is prepared and equipped to hear and respond. Clearly, Shirley's pastor was not prepared or equipped and his counsel probably endangered her further.

The second question is what is the victim/survivor or the abuser disclosing? As was described above, there are at least two possible circumstances: Intimate partner violence which includes sexual violence, but also intimate relationships that do not include a pattern of coercive control (enforced by physical threat and violence) but rely on the assumption of sexual access by the male to the female in the context of entitlement.

In the first instance, the disclosure of IPV or domestic violence, including sexual assault, means that the faith leader should hear, believe, name the danger of the situation, and refer to domestic violence resources in the community with the priority being safety for the victim/survivor. In this case, do not recommend couples' counseling nor contact the abuser without the victim's consent and assurance that she is safe. An excellent resource is Al Miles's *Domestic violence: What every pastor needs to know* (2011). If the faith leader has the opportunity to confront the abuser (either because he has been arrested and is in jail or because he has disclosed and is confessional), then I recommend Carol Adams's narrative:

> What should Shirley's minister have done? He should have said to her rapist, "You have just told me that you broke a law. You have also violated the church's most basic ethical position on covenantal relationships. Will you call the police or shall I?" This offers the opportunity to say to the assailant, "What you did was wrong. You need to get counseling to learn more appropriate ways of responding. I know that court-ordered counseling is often the only way that perpetrators actually participate fully in the counseling program. Through the prosecution for your offense, you are being offered the chance to change, to learn more effect-ive ways of interacting, and to respect your partner. I will support you in this."
>
> (Adams, 1993, p. 75)

In other words, the faith leader's role is to stand by the victim/survivor and call the abuser to account. The only hope of healing the brokenness of this relationship is through change on the part of the abuser.

If, however, the victim/survivor discloses coercive sexual intimacy seemingly assumed by the partner as "normal" but experienced by the victim/survivor as nonconsensual, then the faith leader's response is first to affirm and support the disclosure, and, with her permission, confront the assumption on the husband's part that he is entitled to sexual access to his wife without her consent. Faith leaders should draw on the resources of their faith tradition to support their discussion (see above) and have resources available for referral if the couple wishes to address their sexual relationship together.

## Conclusion

What we are seeing here in the intersection of faith traditions and IPSV is historically two failures. First is the failure to see and name IPV that is occurring within each of our faith communities and too often with the tacit approval of faith leaders. The second failure is the inadequacy of our various versions of sexual ethics which have neglected the fundamental principle of authentic consent as necessary for healthy sexual intimacy in marriage or any sexual relationship.

It is the primary responsibility of faith leaders and scholars within our various traditions to name IPSV as contrary to the fundamental values and teachings of our various traditions, and to confront the misuse and misappropriation of sacred texts and teachings. Faith and religion are certainly part of the problem of domestic and sexual violence, but they can make a significant contribution to the solution. In our various faith communities, we need an open and forthright discussion of authentic consent in all sexual relationships, including marriage. This means preaching and teaching to create a public discussion to encourage change of the cultural norms which have allowed IPSV to go on for centuries. Providing this context then allows us to clearly confront IPSV as antithetical to a healthy, intimate relationship and to draw on the values of our faith traditions to support couples and families.

## References

Abrahamson, A. (1996, January 29). Defendant says he has right to sex with wife. *Los Angeles Times.*

Abugideiri, S., & Magid, M. (2014). *Before you tie the knot: A guide for couples.* Publisher: Createspace Independent Publishing, Authors.

Adams, Carol J. (1993). "I just raped my wife! What are you going to do about it, Pastor?": The Church and sexual violence. In E. Buchwald, P.R. Fletcher, & M. Roth (Eds.), *Transforming a rape culture.* Minneapolis, MN: Milkweed Editions.

Allen, B. (2008, June 27). Southern Baptist scholar links spouse abuse to wives' refusal to submit to their husbands. Retrieved from the Ethics Daily website, www.ethicsdaily.com/

southern-baptist-scholar-links-spouse-abuse-to-wives-refusal-to-submit-to-their-husbands-cms-12832.

Anne, L. (2012, July 19). Marital rape? Doug Wilson on dominance and submission in the marriage bed. Retrieved from the Patheos website: www.patheos.com/blogs/lovejoy feminism/2012/07/marital-rape-doug-wilson-on-dominance-and-submission-in-the-marriage-bed.html.

Cooper-White, P. (1995). *The cry of Tamar: Violence against women and the Church's response.* Minneapolis, MN: Fortress Press.

Davidson, T. (1978). *Conjugal crime.* New York, NY: Hawthorn Books.

Dratch, M. (2014). I do? Consent and coercion in sexual relations. In L.J. Grushcow (Ed.), *The sacred encounter: Jewish perspectives on sexuality.* New York, NY: CCAR Press.

Driscoll, Mark (2014) Pastor Mark Driscoll called women "penis homes." Retrieved from: www.patheos.com/blogs/lovejoyfeminism/2014/09/pastor-mark-driscoll-called-women-penis-homes.html.

Fortune, Marie M. (1983). *Sexual violence: The unmentionable sin. An ethical and pastoral perspective.* Cleveland, OH: The Pilgrim Press.

Fortune, Marie M. (1987). *Keeping the faith: Guidance for Christian women facing abuse.* New York, NY: HarperOne.

Fortune, Marie M. (1995). *Love does no harm: Sexual ethics for the rest of us.* New York, NY: Continuum Publishing Co.

Gruenenfelder, J.B. (1972). The unity of the marital act. In M.J. Taylor (Ed.), *Sex: Thoughts for contemporary Christians.* New York, NY: Doubleday & Co.

Guernsey, Henry N. (1882). *Plain talks on avoided subjects.* Philadelphia, PA: F.A. Davis.

Miles, A. (2011). *Domestic violence: What every pastor needs to know.* Minneapolis, MN: Fortress Press.

Rich, A. (1979). *On lies, secrets, and silence: Selected prose 1966–1978.* New York, NY: W.W. Norton.

Yllo, K., & LeClerc, D. (1988). Marital rape. In A.L. Horton & J.A. Williamson (Eds.), *Abuse and religion.* New York, NY: D.C. Heath & Co.

*Biblical texts cited are from the New Revised Standard Version, 1989 (NRSV).*

# Part 5

# Community prevention and intervention with perpetrators

# Chapter 17

# Addressing and combating intimate partner sexual violence

*Rus Ervin Funk and Lundy Bancroft*

Intimate partner sexual violence (IPSV) is a complex problem that has severe implications for interpersonal relationships and women's health and well-being, in addition to broader social consequences related to gender equality, women's human rights generally, and reproductive and sexual justice. Working to intervene with men who perpetrate IPSV requires that such intervention be done with men in the context of these broader social consequences. As critical as it is, it is not enough for interventionists to work solely to manage individual perpetrators, or to help men become less likely to reoffend. Interventionists must work in concert with other social justice advocates and activists, on this issue and others, to help make the social change necessary to prevent intimate partner sexual violence from occurring in the first place.

Male perpetration of IPSV occurs in a context in which women's sexuality is commodified and objectified. Women, in general, are undervalued vis-à-vis men. Sexuality, particularly women's sexuality, is restricted and problematized. For example, comprehensive and sex-positive sexuality education is limited or nonexistent (Guttmacher Institute, 2016). Along with numerous colleagues in the field, both of us believe – based on evidence from experience working in the field – that intervening with men who perpetrate intimate partner sexual violence without addressing these other factors has minimal effect. While we may be successful in reducing an individual's likelihood to reoffend, we do nothing to address or shift the broader social context that creates each next generation of men who perpetrate IPSV.

In this chapter, we explore some of the factors associated with male perpetration of IPSV, outline strategies for practitioners to work across many of these factors, and explore what a comprehensive intervention might look like. Together, we have more than 50 years' experience working with men who perpetrate sexual and intimate partner violence, and working at the community level to prevent all forms of gender-based violence (GBV).

## Common misconceptions regarding the causes of sexual offending

In order to intervene with sexual assault perpetrators, service providers need to base their work in a realistic understanding of where the exploitative behaviors stem from. There is a tendency to settle on one of two extreme perspectives in viewing the perpetrator, both of which are problematic. Both tend to focus on the individual as the sole source of the behavior.

One extreme is to view the perpetrator as someone who simply doesn't understand what appropriate behavior is and who misreads cues. From this view, the perpetrator doesn't need a punitive response; he just needs some clear education about boundaries and about consent, and then he won't make the same mistake again. This perspective seems to be an especially tempting one when the perpetrator is popular or is a valued member of his community – for example, as an athlete, educator, or faith leader (Edwards, 2013; Sander, 2007). It lends itself regrettably well to circumstances where the community doesn't want to believe that he committed the offense, or wants to see it as a product of some kind of misunderstanding. The problematic outcomes of this view are several, including:

- The perpetrator who doesn't experience uncomfortable consequences for his actions is unlikely to change.
- In the absence of consequences, counseling and educational interventions for perpetrators are known to be largely ineffective, though research suggests that they do have some effectiveness when used *in combination with* meaningful strong consequences (Gondolf, 2002).
- Skepticism may increase in response to future reports from victims of the same man, as people feel that "he dealt with his issues" and that therefore the new report is unlikely to be true.
- Lack of systemic structures and processes of accountability means leaving these men to their own devices to figure out how not to get caught the next time.

The other extreme perspective is to see the sexual assault perpetrator as a monster, a person devoid of all human feeling, full of hatred and violence, who hides behind bushes or who drives up and forces victims into his car. Services for this man would be seen as pointless, and the goal would be to take the most punitive action possible. This view is actually no less dangerous to victims of sexual assault than the one we described above, for the following reasons:

1. Most sexual assault perpetrators do not fit this "monster" profile (although a few will) with the result that the great majority will tend to escape accountability because they won't be perceived as the "real" offender type.

2. This view has the effect of miseducating women about warning signs to watch for, thereby increasing their vulnerability to assault. (For example, the sexual assault perpetrator will more commonly come in a smooth, charming package than in the form of an obvious hostile threat.)

3. Although jailing perpetrators and imposing other kinds of consequences are important measures, they will very often not lead to lasting changes in the man's behavior. We need to find ways to get services to all perpetrators.

4. "Accountability" here is seen as the exclusive purview of the criminal legal system, relieving the rest of us of any responsibility to challenge the perpetrator in his behavior.

We believe that there is a need for a more nuanced and comprehensive view of the sexual assault perpetrator – both in general and specifically men who perpetrate intimate partner sexual violence. Because he may be perceived to be an upstanding member of the community, we can't simply demonize him; on the other hand, we can't minimize the depth and seriousness of his problems, even with a first-time offender. Further, we consider it crucial to understand the process by which he developed into a man willing to perpetrate violence and abuse toward women. This development takes place in a broader context. The attitudes and perspectives that reinforce his perpetrating behaviors have been supported and encouraged at multiple layers: friends, family and colleagues, social norms, and community values.

Effectively intervening means not only addressing his individual rationale for perpetrating sexual violence, but preparing him to manage the collusion he has received and will continue to receive from various key players at these levels. Better still, intervention with perpetrators of IPSV should be nested within current broader social change efforts that work to challenge and counter these layers of support that men receive to perpetrate violence and abuse. The ideal end result would be that intervention with men who perpetrate IPSV exists within a dynamic movement designed to eliminate the option for any men to ever perpetrate such violence.

Intimate partner sexual violence can be best understood as a subset of sexual violence overall. And men who perpetrate intimate partner sexual violence can be seen as a subset of sexual assault perpetrators. Therefore, misperceptions about sexual assault perpetrators have particular manifestations within the context of intimate partner relationships. As Ricardo and Barker (2008, p. 21) state: "Understandings of sexual violence are particularly complicated in the context of intimate relationships where perceptions of women's consent and men's entitlement are often confused or unclear, on the part of both men and women (and in many national laws)." In short, IPSV has particular and additional factors that contribute to its perpetration.

We tend to view a husband who rapes his wife as either a poorly misunderstood, probably sexually frustrated man who doesn't know a better way to get his needs met, or as a complete bully who uses sexual violence in the context of other forms of violence and control within the relationship to dominate and humiliate his partner. Neither view provides an effective pathway for intervention, due to the failure to address the specific entitled attitudes, belief in ownership over females, view of sexuality as conquest, and other dynamics of coercive control that play such a central role in IPSV.

As Ricardo and Barker (2008) suggest, entitlement is one of the core factors contributing to men's perpetration of intimate partner sexual violence. Men are not born with a sense of entitlement to women's bodies in general, and their wives or girlfriends in particular. Men *learn* both that they are entitled to have sex with someone else – particularly a partner – and the specific ways to assert/enforce this sense of entitlement through multiple means. It is an entitlement that is reinforced across what Bronfenbrenner (1976) describes as the "social ecology." He suggests, and others (see for example, Funk, 2005; Jewkes, Flood, & Lang, 2015; Douglas et al., 2008) have developed this, that effective intervention requires work across the whole of the social ecology. Ultimately, if our goal is to end IPSV, working with men who perpetrate as a means to address these large social factors is a critical aspect of the work which, by and large, still needs to be developed.

## What it takes to perpetrate sexual assault

From a variety of sources, including victim accounts, research studies, and confessed perpetrators, we know that a great deal has to occur before a man harms a female in a sexual way, particularly a female he claims to love. What we refer to below is taken from the collective knowledge in regard to sexual assault perpetrators in general, of which IPSV perpetrators can be conceived of as a subset. While we don't necessarily reference IPSV in each of these areas below, what we're describing refers to perpetrators of sexual violence more broadly as well as to perpetrators of IPSV. Specifically:

1.  He has to develop an inordinate lack of empathy for the woman's feelings (Lisak & Ivan, 1995; Simons, Wurtele, & Heil, 2002). Although the perpetrator often claims that he had no idea that his behavior was causing her distress, the reality is that her lack of consent is obvious (as confessed perpetrators commonly admit) (Scully, 2013; Scully & Marolla, 1993). In order to harm someone in a sexual way, he has to have developed an internal process that allows him to decide that her pain doesn't count, that the long-term harm to her won't exist or doesn't matter, and that her lack of consent is irrelevant. In short, his blocks to empathy are huge.

    This lack of empathy is not natural. The social ecology framework provides a model to explore how someone develops this lack of empathy and as such, suggests an intervention approach that is necessary in order to reestablish this empathy with others.

2.   He has to construct an elaborate system of justifications for his behavior. The perpetrator has to live with what he has done, and in order to do so he has to persuade himself that exploiting women sexually is acceptable, that he is not responsible for his actions, and that women are beneath him. Further, he has to come to believe that lying to her, about her, and about his own actions are all excusable choices.

Intervening with men who perpetrate IPSV includes examining how their system of justification is established (so that it can be deconstructed), and how their construction of a system of justification is reinforced across the social ecology.

3.   He has to envision sexual assault (including in most cases envisioning an assault against this specific victim – in IPSV, his partner). A majority of sexual assaults are planned; and even for those that were not planned, we have good reason to believe (based on accounts of confessed perpetrators) that the man had long experience of imagining what he might do to a woman and becoming enamored of those images.

DeKeseredy and Schwartz (2013) show how male peers support this kind of imagining and enamoring of sexual violence, and one needs only look at media images to see countless examples of this kind of imagery (see Chapters 13 and 14 for further discussion of social support of IPSV).

4.   He has to feel a significant degree of social approval for his actions prior to committing them. (This is especially true of the more common, less monstrous, type of offender.) Sexual assault perpetrators learn justifications and strategies, and the mentality that allows them to block out the feelings and humanity of their victims, from various social sources. These include influences within the home (sexual assault perpetrators come disproportionately from homes where their father or another male in the home battered their mother); peer relationships, especially during their teenage years; violent pornography; and other sources (DeKeseredy & Corsianos, 2016).

5.   He has to trust that his actions will be unlikely to be found out, and if they are, that he will not be held accountable for his behaviors in any significant ways.

As described above, these factors (and others) associated with male perpetration of IPSV (understood here as a subset of sexual violence) can be located on the social ecology and provide a further framework for effective intervention efforts. Recognizing the ways that multiple factors across the social ecology support these belief systems, interventionists are better able to work with men who perpetrate in ways that both counter these messages *and* can work to help undermine these factors. In this way, intervention efforts can become more effectively preventionist.

Examining some of the contributing factors, across the social ecology, which contribute to men's perpetration of IPSV suggests the following (Figure 17.1). (Please note: this is not meant as an exhaustive list of the contributing factors at each level, but rather a snapshot for the purposes of this chapter.)

- *On the individual level*: Sense of entitlement, having been sexually or physically abused himself, rigid and traditional gender roles, pornography use, perpetration of domestic violence.
- *On the relational level*: Exposure to domestic violence as a child, having a close relationship with a father or father figure who held rigid gender roles, having a peer network that supports his attitudes if not his actual behavior.
- *At the community level*: Gender inequality, lack of comprehensive and accessible sexuality education, prevalence of victim-blaming, nonexistent or inconsistent community sanctions against gender-based violence.
- *At the social level*: Lack of social or legal sanctions against IPSV, gender inequality, media images that promote male dominance and aggression and which promote victim-blaming.

Effective intervention with men who perpetrate IPSV focuses on their individual behaviors in the context of these other factors. Working solely with the individual who perpetrates IPSV (if that is in individual treatment or in a group context) is not sufficient as an intervention strategy. Working with individual men in the context of their peer networks, community, and the broader social environment is also necessary.

## Toward solutions: A comprehensive approach

We see practitioners working with men who perpetrate IPSV as (at least potentially) on the front lines of our global work toward gender respect, gender equality, and gender justice. Aldarondo (2007) provides multiple examples of ways that practitioners, working clinically, can help promote broader social justice goals. Evidence and experience suggest that in environments that are respectful, equitable, and just, the perpetration of intimate partner and sexual violence is reduced significantly. Although no one, to our knowledge, has specifically examined the relationship of a just and equitable social environment to the perpetration of IPSV, it would seem self-evident that this is the case. In these kinds of environments, efforts to work with, hold accountable, and help rehabilitate men who perpetrate IPSV are imbedded in robust comprehensive efforts to prevent all forms of gender-based violence and promote gender equity and gender justice more broadly.

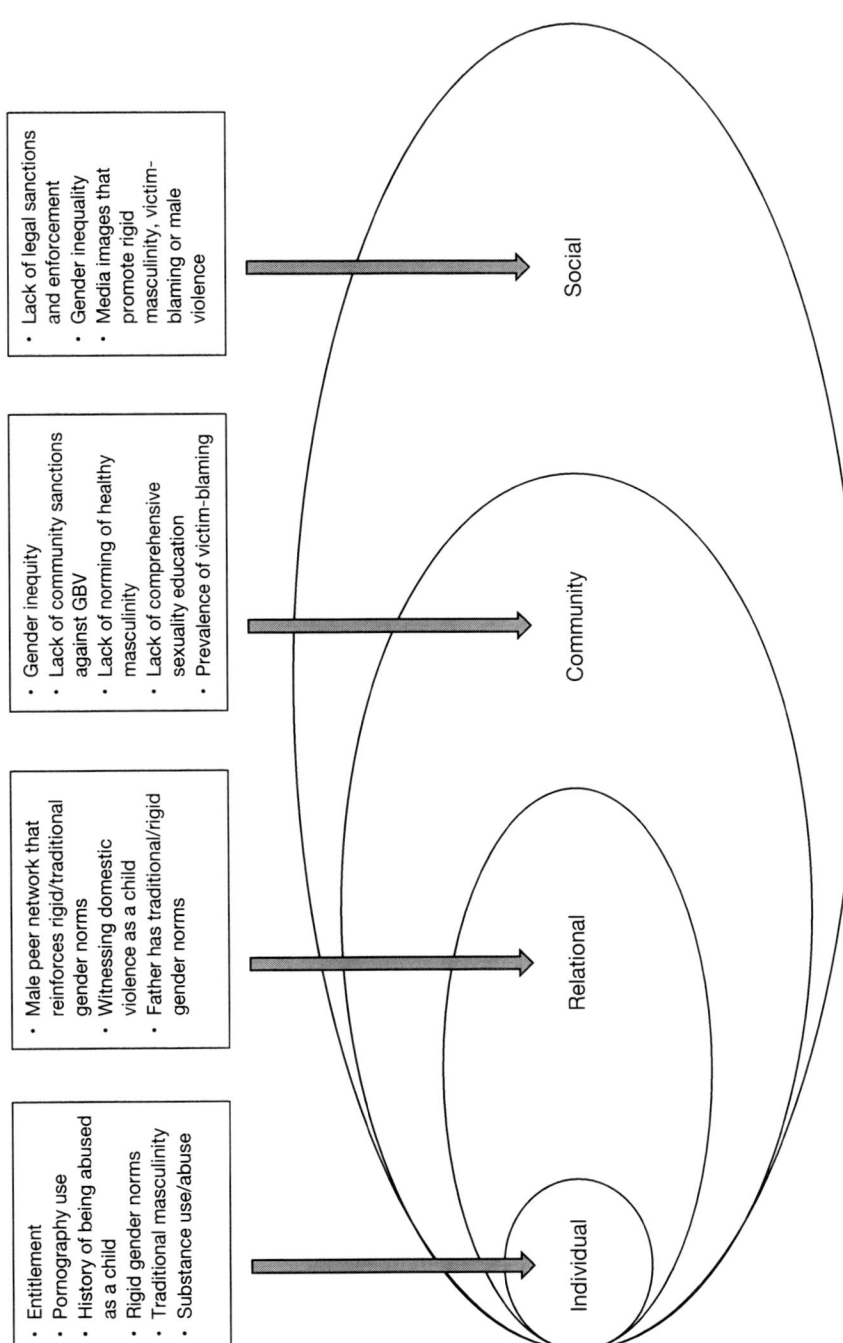

- Entitlement
- Pornography use
- History of being abused as a child
- Rigid gender norms
- Traditional masculinity
- Substance use/abuse

- Male peer network that reinforces rigid/traditional gender norms
- Witnessing domestic violence as a child
- Father has traditional/rigid gender norms

- Gender inequity
- Lack of community sanctions against GBV
- Lack of norming of healthy masculinity
- Lack of comprehensive sexuality education
- Prevalence of victim-blaming

- Lack of legal sanctions and enforcement
- Gender inequality
- Media images that promote rigid masculinity, victim-blaming or male violence

Individual

Relational

Community

Social

*Figure 17.1* Factors across the social ecology contributing to men's perpetration of intimate partner sexual violence

From this perspective, working solely with individuals to promote gender respect, then releasing them into an ocean of gender disrespect and devaluing of women, may undo their progress in intervention groups. The work being done around the world to engage men in the prevention of gender-based violence is instructive. Based on the emerging data, working with men across the social ecology is proving, by leaps and bounds, to be most effective in shifting individuals' support for gender equality, enhancing social norms that promote gender equality, and changing community values and political support for gender equality (USAID, 2015; World Health Organization, 2007; Wells, et al., 2013).

## Implications for intervention with IPSV perpetrators

The object of describing these preconditions in such detail is to make it clear that intervening to stop IPSV perpetrators from reoffending are necessarily part of a large and serious project. It is a fallacy to think that some brief education and counseling are going to have any significant effect. In order to have a meaningful impact, interventions will need to include:

1.  Serious, unwelcome consequences for the perpetrator, both to dissuade him from reoffending and to increase his motivation to participate seriously in sexual offender services.
2.  Services that address the full range of issues we laid out in the four points above regarding the preconditions of perpetration.
3.  Services that are of long enough duration to be able to realistically foster change, given the length of process that is involved (generally viewed as in the range of 18 months to 3 years) to make lasting attitudinal and behavioral changes.
4.  Service providers who will not be misled by the perpetrator's mild social persona, his convincing minimizations and distortions of his actions, and his victim-blaming.

Addressing sexual violence must be included in all programs and efforts working with men who batter. Sexual violence should be both a specific topic that is addressed, *and* content that is incorporated as an aspect of the coercive control tactics or abuse behaviors used by men who batter. It is safe to assume that the overwhelming majority of men who perpetrate intimate partner violence have also utilized some of these abusive tactics with respect to the sexual aspect of their intimate relationship. They may have used one or more sexual assaults as part of their violence tactics, but sexual violence within a relationship can also include demanding sex after a violent attack, forcing their partner to perform what they have viewed on pornography (with or without actual threats), demeaning their partner's sexuality or sexual "performance," or having other sexual partners and ensuring that their partner knows about these other encounters or relationships. Abused women, their advocates, and scholars have raised concerns about the difficulty of defining any sex as consensual in the context of intimidation that abuse creates; in the words of one study, "Battered women know what they risk if they refuse the sexual advances of the batterer" (Mahoney & Williams, 1998, p. 130).

In intervention with men who batter, questions that explore the forms of coercion, manipulation, and force that they may have used in order to be sexual with their partner need to be a part of the assessment and the intervention (see Chapter 8 for additional information on the various forms of IPSV). For example, exploring their understanding of the difference between seduction and coercion is one strategy for assessing their perpetration of IPSV within the relationship. The degree to which the individual cannot distinguish between these two, is the degree to which a focus on IPSV should be incorporated as a part of that person's intervention process.

Since male peer support is a significant contributing factor to men's perpetration of domestic violence, sexual violence in general, and IPSV in particular, addressing this within an intervention strategy is a critical aspect of the intervention. In intervention groups, participants can learn how to develop new peer networks that hold values of gender respect, gender equality, and healthy sexuality; they can learn how to create peer networks of accountability; and they can learn to integrate their current peer networks into their process of becoming nonviolent and respectful within their relationships. These skills and concepts are critical to effective intervention models with men who perpetrate.

One example of just such a process comes from Men Stopping Violence in Atlanta. Their intervention strategy involves several sessions that include peer networks as identified by the men in the program (Douglass, Bathrick, & Perry, 2008). The client must bring a subset of his peer network to several sessions (the same peer network) in order for them to learn how to support him in his path toward nonviolence and gender respect. This model seems like a relatively easy addition to current intervention strategies that begin reaching out into the social ecology, and one that most intervention practitioners would implement.

Men who perpetrate can be encouraged and supported, as a part of their participation, to plan an event or program to combat intimate partner violence or promote gender equality community-wide. Consider the learning potential of having men, as a part of their intervention, design a community-wide "men's march against domestic violence." As a part of a group that Rus Funk led, participants were required to create and present an educational workshop to adolescent men about rape, sexual assault, sexual respect or some related topic (under the close supervision of Rus and the local rape crisis center). Using the tool "we all learn best when we start to teach," this experience proved a powerful learning opportunity for the men in the group, as well as a way for Rus to differently assess how they were doing in learning and integrating the content of the group.

Men who are in a group process to address their perpetration of IPSV can also be mobilized to challenge some of the media images that have fueled their justifications for perpetrating sexual violence in the first place. This kind of strategy helps them to develop some critical media skills that can assist them in their recovery (i.e. how to continue to consume media while also challenging some of the socially negative and destructive messaging and social norming that exist within those media). It can also begin to empower men individually and as a collective to have a voice to make social change. The experience of the ways in which working for social change contributes to the healing process for people who have been victimized (Herman, 1992) suggests the potential value of these same strategies to help men who perpetrate to make amends in a different way, and be more accountable.

## Concluding thoughts

Working to effectively combat intimate partner sexual violence requires our working across the social ecology and at the intersections of IPSV with other social problems. It requires individual change efforts married with broader social change movements. And it requires that we, whoever "we" may be, work in collaboration with other partners to make these connections and to do what is necessary to promote relationships that never include sexual violence.

## References

Aldarondo, E. (2007). *Advancing social justice through clinical practice*. New York, NY: Routledge.

Bronfenbrenner, U. (1976). *The ecology of human development: Experiments by nature and design*. Cambridge, MA: Harvard University Press.

DeKeseredy, W.S., & Corsianos, M. (2016). *Violence against women in pornography*. New York, NY: Routledge Press.

DeKeseredy W.S., & Schwartz, M. (2013) *Male peer support and violence against women: The history and verification of a theory*. Boston, MA: Northeastern University Press.

Douglas, U., Bathrick, D., & Perry, P.A. (2008). Deconstructing male violence against women. *Violence Against Women, 14*(2), 247–261.

Edwards, D. (2013). CNN grieves that guilty verdict ruined "promising" lives of Steubenville rapists. Retrieved from: www.rawstory.com/2013/03/cnn-grieves-that-guilty-verdict-ruined-promising-lives-of-steubenville-rapists/.

Funk, R.E. (2005). *Reaching men: Strategies for preventing sexist attitudes, behaviors and violence*. Indianapolis, IN: Jist Publications.

Gondolf, E. (2002). *Batterer intervention systems*. Thousand Oaks, CA: Sage Publications.

Guttmacher Institute (2016). American teens' sources of sexual health education. Retrieved from: www.guttmacher.org/fact-sheet/facts-american-teens-sources-information-about-sex.

Herman, J. (1992). *Trauma and recovery*. New York, NY: Basic Books.

Jewkes, R., Flood, M., & Lang, J. (2015). From work with men and boys to changes of social norms and reduction of inequities in gender relations: A conceptual shift in prevention of violence against women and girls. *The Lancet, 385*(9977), 1580–1589. http://dx/doi.org/10.1016/S0140–6736(14)61683-4.

Lisak, D., & Ivan, C. (1995). Deficits in intimacy and empathy in sexually aggressive men. *Journal of Interpersonal Violence, 10*(3), 296–308.

Mahoney, P., & Williams, L.M. (1998). Sexual assault in marriage: Prevalence, consequences, and treatment of wife rape. In J. Jasinski & L.M. Williams (Eds.), *Partner violence: A comprehensive review of 20 years of research* (pp. 113–163). Thousand Oaks, CA: Sage Publications.

Ricardo, C., & Barker, G. (2008). Men, masculinities, sexual exploitation and sexual violence: A literature review and call for action. Global MenEngage Alliance. Retrieved from: http://menengage.org/resources/men-masculinities-sexual-exploitation-sexual-violence-literature-review-call-action-2/.

Sander, L. (2007). U. of Colorado at Boulder settles lawsuit over alleged rapes at football recruiting party for $2.85 million. Retrieved from: www.titleix.info/resources/Legal-Cases/Colorado-Lawsuit-Alleged-Rape-Football-Recruiting-Party.aspx.

Scully, D. (2013). *Understanding sexual violence: A study of convicted rapists.* New York, NY: Routledge.

Scully, D., & Marolla, J. (1993). "Riding the bull at Gilley's": Convicted rapists describe the rewards of rape. In P.B. Bart and E.G. Moran (Eds.), *Violence against women: The bloody footprints* (pp. 26–46). Thousand Oaks, CA: Sage.

Simons, D., Wurtele, S.K., & Heil, P. (2002). Childhood victimization and lack of empathy as predictors of sexual offending against women and children. *Journal of Interpersonal Violence, 17*(12), 1291–1307.

USAID (2015). Working with men and boys to end violence against women and girls: Approaches, challenges and lessons. Retrieved from the USAID website: www.usaid.gov/sites/default/files/Sector-2-%20Education_MenandBoys.pdf.

Wells, L., Lorenzetti, L., Carolo, H., Dinner, T., Jones, C., Minerson, T., & Esina, E. (2013). *Engaging men and boys in domestic violence prevention: Opportunities and promising approaches. Shift: The project to end domestic violence.* Calgary, Canada: University of Calgary.

World Health Organization (2007). Engaging men and boys in changing gender-based inequity in health: Evidence from programme interventions. Retrieved from: www.who.int/gender/documents/Engaging_men_boys.pdf.

# Chapter 18

# Intimate partner sexual violence and perpetrator programs

## Project Mirabal research findings

*Nicole Westmarland and Liz Kelly*

## Introduction

There is far more research on sex offender treatment programs – programs specifically for those convicted of sexual offenses – than there is known about the use of sexual violence by men in domestic violence perpetrator programs (DVPPs, known as batterer intervention programs in the US). However, given the widespread nature of sexual violence within domestic violence, it is clear that this is an important topic for DVPPs to be addressing.

This chapter begins with a description of how one DVPP addresses sexual violence drawing on their course materials. It then presents findings from Project Mirabal, an investigation of the contribution of DVPPs, using quantitative data on whether sexual violence continued after the program and qualitative interview data to explore how the men on programs and women partners, and ex-partners talked about sexual violence. Here three themes are discussed: men's use of sexual violence before they went on the program (expectations of sex, pressure); sexual violence histories and herstories (previous experiences of sexual violence and the importance of pornography); and finally accounts of changes made/seen since attending the DVPP.

## Project Mirabal

Project Mirabal was a program of research that considered what domestic violence perpetrator programs add to a coordinated community response in the UK (Kelly & Westmarland, 2015). Innovatively, we linked a pilot study (see Westmarland, Kelly, & Chalder-Mills, 2010 and Westmarland & Kelly, 2013 for more detailed discussion) on what counted as success to four groups of stakeholders (women survivors, men on programs, staff and funders/ commissioners) with Evan Stark's (2007) contention that coercive control concerns not just women's safety but also their freedom. This resulted in six measures of success:

1. Improved relationship based on respect and effective communication.
2. Expanded "space for action" for women.

3.  Safety and freedom from violence and abuse.
4.  Safe, positive and shared parenting.
5.  Enhanced awareness of self and others for men.
6.  Safer, healthier childhoods.

In contrast to other studies on this topic, we collected both quantitative and qualitative data. The quantitative survey was undertaken five times, covering time periods from before the men started on the program to 12 months after the program start date. We also collected survey data on the above six measures from 100 women whose partners attended DVPPs.

In-depth interviews were conducted with 64 men and 48 women partners and ex-partners near the beginning (Time 1) and end (Time 2) of the program. In the interviews, the measures of success were explored in detail. A specific example was chosen by each interviewee who was asked to talk about actions and reactions, what was said, thought, and felt at the time and later.

A specific question about sexual violence was asked within the survey but not within the interviews. Hence, our qualitative analysis consists of data where participants themselves raised the issue of sexual violence within one of the examples we asked about. Data were obtained by searching the entire qualitative data set for relevant search terms (rape, sex, forced).

The participants were self-selecting – mostly white British, in (or previously in) heterosexual relationships – reflecting the current profile of men attending programs. All were drawn from 12 Respect-accredited "community based" domestic violence perpetrator programs in England, Scotland, and Wales. Respect, a UK membership organization, sets program standards which must be met for accreditation. These programs are separate from the criminal justice system and men are not mandated by a criminal court to attend (see Philips, Kelly and Westmarland 2014 for a Project Mirabal paper on the history of perpetrator work in the UK). At the present time, the community-based programs receive most referrals from Children's Services, Children and Family Court Advisory and Support Services (CAFCASS) linked to disputed child contact cases, and local authorities. While some referral routes mean that it is mostly working-class men who attend, the CAFCASS route is less social-class based. Ethical approval for the study was granted by London Metropolitan University.

## What does a sexual violence module within a domestic violence perpetrator program look like?

First, it is important to understand how DVPPs address sexual violence within their programs. Respect-accredited DVPPs – such as the ones in our study – do not have a common, universally agreed upon "manual." Thus, they vary in terms of their content and theoretical perspectives, depending on which (if any) manual they are using as their base; the skills, knowledge, and experience of their facilitators; and the characteristics of the group of men they are working with. That said, the topic of sexual respect was a core component covered in all of the programs involved in Project Mirabal.

The largest DVPP in England is based in London and is called the Domestic Violence Intervention Project (DVIP). The DVIP men's group work program lasts for 26 sessions, usually held weekly, with each session lasting two-and-a-half hours. The sexual respect and abuse module consists of material from their core manual and more recent material developed as part of the Jacana Parenting Program (see Coy et al., 2011 for evaluation). Facilitators also develop additional materials in response to any identified gaps.

This module is described as intended to:

- help men move away from the taboo of discussing sex honestly and seriously;
- increase empathy and understanding of women's perspectives rather than focusing solely on the men's own sense of entitlement around sex;
- recognize the benefits of sexually respectful relationships;
- learn how to negotiate and communicate with their partners around establishing a sexually respectful relationship.

(DVIP, 2010)

The manual notes that exercises used will vary from group to group but might include small group discussions to consider how participants developed their beliefs and expectations around sex and how these might differ from other people's, including their partners, as well as more specific discussions around what is meant by sexual abuse and its effects on women. A written scenario may be used to ask group members to identify where sexual abuse starts, with the aim being recognition that relying only on legal definitions can overlook a range of sexually coercive, pressuring behaviors.

Box 18.1 presents one of the written scenarios used by DVIP.

---

### Box 18.1 Sexual abuse scenario: "Paul and Lisa"

Paul and Lisa have been together for three years. Initially, they had sex frequently, but now she's often not in the mood and Paul feels she has to be coaxed.

On the night in question Paul brings her home some flowers. Later, they are sitting together watching TV and Paul starts to be affectionate with her. He puts his arm around her, tells her she looks great and kisses her. Then he begins trying to get sexual with her by touching her breasts. She pushes him away, gives a little laugh and says, "You're incorrigible!".

He says, "Come on sweetheart, I'm just messing around," and tries again to kiss her. Now she pulls away again, still smiling, and tells him, "Not now, I'm tired, I'm just not in the mood."

Paul says, "But we haven't made love for ages and I just want to show you I love you" and once again tries to kiss her. She is now not smiling. She pushes him away and says more firmly, "No, I said I don't feel like it."

Paul asks, "Why? What's wrong with me?", but Lisa just replies, "Look, I just don't feel like it, OK?"

For a while Paul questions Lisa about her not loving him any more. He asks her if she's seeing someone else and she tells him not to be silly, but otherwise she is generally unresponsive. Paul mutters that he might as well get it somewhere else for all Lisa seems to care. He moves away and begins to sulk.

Finally she goes to bed. Paul continues to watch TV for a while and then goes up to bed. He wakes her by kissing and touching her. She is initially unresponsive but he badgers and touches her some more, and finally she stops protesting and they have sex.

*Source:* DVIP (2010) *Jacana Parenting Program Manual*, p. 174.

The facilitators then draw a continuum on a flipchart/whiteboard which ranges from "consensual activity" to "violent rape" and the men are asked to identify at what point, if at all, Paul crosses the line between consensual activity and rape. This is shown in Box 18.2.

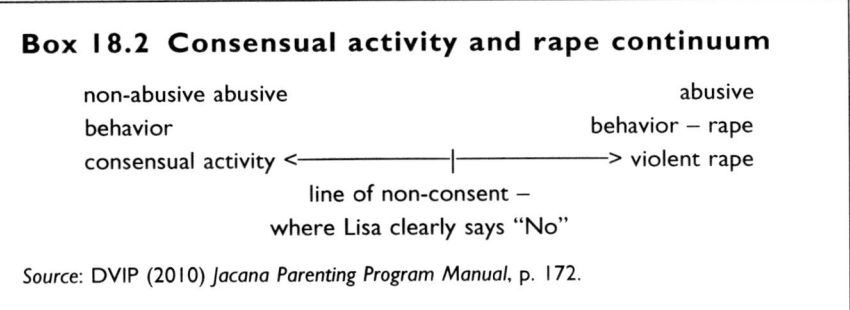

**Box 18.2 Consensual activity and rape continuum**

| non-abusive abusive | abusive |
| behavior | behavior – rape |

consensual activity <————————|————————> violent rape

line of non-consent –
where Lisa clearly says "No"

*Source:* DVIP (2010) *Jacana Parenting Program Manual*, p. 172.

Discussion is then steered toward talking about how Paul might not have crossed the line of continuing once Lisa had clearly said "no," but that his behaviors can still be classed as abusive. This leads to the learning point that the model in Box 18.2 is inadequate because of its focus on an assumption of consent rather than on finding out whether Lisa is genuinely and actively consenting. An alternative model is suggested based on "receptiveness" rather than "consent" as illustrated in Box 18.3.

---

**Box 18. 3 An alternative model based on receptiveness**

Receptive, non-abusive

receptive/active <————————————————> receptive/passive

Non-receptive, abusive

coercion <————————————————> violent rape

Source: DVIP (2010) *Jacana Parenting Program Manual*, p. 173

---

The men are asked to reconsider Paul's behavior along this new continuum, and the role of the facilitator is to show that Paul is on the abusive continuum almost from the start of the scenario (depending on whether the gift of flowers is read as part of the coercion – i.e. whether or not there were "strings attached" to the giving of the flowers). The aim of the exercise is to show that any nonreceptive sexual advances are on the abusive continuum, even if they are some way from "violent rape."

## Project mirabal: Key quantitative findings on physical and sexual violence

We now move onto the findings from the quantitative part of Project Mirabal – focusing on the questions that relate to physical and sexual violence (see Kelly and Westmarland, 2015, for more detailed findings). Figure 18.1 presents the quantitative data for the indicators on the violence and abuse measure of success for "before" (the baseline prior to attending DVPP) and "after" (12 months after starting the program). It shows that all of the physical violence measures decreased substantially, with those for sexual violence decreasing from 30% to nil. Sexual violence in this part of the study was measured through the statement "made you do something sexual that you did not want to do."

This finding suggests that the work undertaken as described in the previous section could give rise to some level of optimism. However, it is important to remember that this is only one question about sexual violence and it does not cover the range of ways men are encouraged to question their expectations and behaviors. It is also important to recognize that some of the women in our sample (around one in six) separated from their partners before, during or

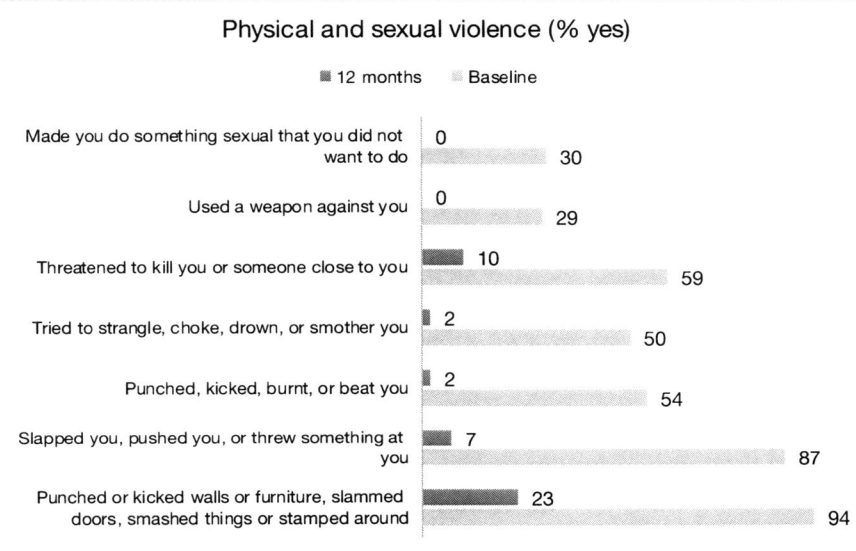

## Physical and sexual violence (% yes)

■ 12 months   ░ Baseline

| | |
|---|---|
| Made you do something sexual that you did not want to do | 0 / 30 |
| Used a weapon against you | 0 / 29 |
| Threatened to kill you or someone close to you | 10 / 59 |
| Tried to strangle, choke, drown, or smother you | 2 / 50 |
| Punched, kicked, burnt, or beat you | 2 / 54 |
| Slapped you, pushed you, or threw something at you | 7 / 87 |
| Punched or kicked walls or furniture, slammed doors, smashed things or stamped around | 23 / 94 |

*Figure 18.1* Physical and sexual violence (% Yes)

after the program – in other words, there may have been fewer opportunities for men to commit the forms of sexual violence that we asked about. It is for these reasons that it is important to consider the quantitative findings alongside those from the in-depth interviews – the ways in which men on programs and their female partners and ex-partners talked about sexual respect (or lack of) within their relationships.

### How men and women talked about sexual violence

As previously noted, there was no specific question about sexual violence asked within the qualitative interviews. This was not an oversight on our part. We developed the interview schedule as a team, attempting to work in a feminist collective way. The issue of sexual violence questions within the qualitative interview schedule was brought up and discussed, but the four researchers who were going to be doing the majority of the interviews were resistant to asking about it. While they did ask about it in the quantitative surveys, these were conducted over the telephone rather than face-to-face, as with the interviews. In addition, a statement reminding the participants that they were free to skip any questions they did not feel comfortable answering preceded the question. This was particularly important given that one of the four researchers was male.

It is debatable, though, whether we were right to leave out a direct question about sexual violence within the qualitative interviews. On one hand, not asking about a form of partner violence can lead to that form being sidelined – as has arguably been seen in the study of this topic and the dearth of academic research on intimate partner sexual violence. On the other hand, we did not ask about other specific forms of partner violence within the qualitative interview. Instead, participants were asked about situations where things did or did not happen, allowing them to talk about the forms of partner violence experienced. It is also important that the researchers asking the questions felt confident with the interview schedules they were using.

On balance, therefore, not asking a specific question was the right judgment call in this study. It does, however, elevate longstanding concerns that we both have about the sidelining of sexual violence within partner violence research and the need to ensure that researchers are trained and feel confident in asking about this. The fact that many of the participants felt able to talk openly about sexual violence in the detailed ways we now present is testament to the skills and abilities, if not confidence, of the Project Mirabal researchers and to the willingness of participants to explore these areas.

The remainder of this chapter consists of a thematic analysis of the interview material where sexual violence was raised within responses to broader questions – particularly those connected to the six measures of success. Pseudonyms are used and the information in parentheses indicates whether the interview was conducted near the start (Time 1) or the end (Time 2) of the program.

## Men's use of sexual violence before they went on the program

Sexual violence was discussed by the participants in a range of ways. At its core was a general *expectation of sex* in terms of the role of women within intimate partner relationships. Sometimes *pressure* was applied if there was reluctance on the part of the woman: such pressure sometimes did and at times did not result in acquiescence. When the more subtle tactics of expectations and pressure were insufficient, physical violence or coercive control might be used, including in some instances rendering the woman unconscious through alcohol. We explore each of these tactics through interview data from men on programs and women partners and ex-partners.

### EXPECTATIONS OF SEX

Both men and women talked about how, before the program, there was an expectation that women would continuously consent to sex. The feelings and "needs" of men were deemed central, regardless of whether these were compatible with what women wanted – a finding in line with much previous research on heterosexual partnerships.

Many of the women at Time 1 talked about feeling as though they were sexual objects, to be there at the beck and call of their partners: "I don't know whether it was just, whether he wanted someone to – I can't even say play with – just be there all the time, just for him, like unconditional" (Sophie). June talked of being treated like a "machine for sex." Delia suggested her partner wanted a wife who was "hot, on tap." Martha recalled the pressure put on her to have sexual intercourse soon after a hysterectomy. This was one of the turning points for her in realizing how marginal her views and opinions had become.

> It had never occurred to me before in that all he was ever bothered about was what he wanted and the fact that I'd had a major op he wasn't concerned about, he just wanted what he wanted. I really didn't give it any more thought than that I just thought, 'Well okay, I'm his wife' and it was always focused on him and he never, ever gave me any thought at all. At the time I just accepted that's the way it was and we carried on.
>
> (Martha, Time 1)

Some men at Time 1 acknowledged that they had failed to consider the situation from the woman's perspective. Kevin acknowledged that the expectation of sexual intercourse was a demand he placed on his partner: "I used to be very sexual, and when confronted with a beautiful woman, well then sometimes you expect it on tap, and I put a lot of pressure on her for that." Don talked about such expectations leading to his partner thinking that it was a wife's "duty" always to be available for sex.

> It got to a point where my wife felt it was her duty as a wife to please the husband, okay, which is wrong it shouldn't be like that . . . and I think to take on that kind of role just to keep the peace I think that's how my wife reacted to that situation.
>
> (Don, Time 1)

What we see here are very traditional notions of heterosexual relationships, with male entitlement at the core.

## THE USE OF "PRESSURE"

Alongside this sense of sexual entitlement came the application of pressure if women failed to comply with men's expectations. Don accepted that applying pressure in relation to sex was one of the key ways that he was abusive before he went on the program. Kevin was keen to distinguish between "forceful controlling" and the tactics that he used to pressure his partner into sexual intercourse. Although he maintains that he never actually "forced" her into sex, he concedes that there were occasions where his partner had to say "no" a few times:

... not − not forceful controlling. I never − never forced myself on her ... [I] tried to get her more open than she'd want to, or sometimes kind of felt that we're − we were having a laugh or getting − but then she said, "Not now, not now" and I'd say "OK." Sometimes she'd have to say "no" more often, but, yeah, I don't think I ever forced myself on her.

(Kevin, Time 1)

Delia recalls pressure being the primary tactic her partner used:

Over the years it's a case of he would push us, I'd pull away, he would push us, I'd pull away, so it's like a push−pull relationship. You know he wants more sex; the more he wants the less I want, and it got to a point where he was pressurising me quite a bit with regards to it. In the end it was just shut up and put up. No violence whatsoever, nothing ... no beating up, no threatening or anything like that but just the pressure, the sexual pressure.

(Delia, Time 1)

This is a somewhat different picture than often painted in domestic violence research, where there is a commonly cited presumption that women "give in" to sex in order to prevent further physical abuse. It is, however, in accord with the continuum of nonconsensual sex that Kelly (1987) found some 30 years ago, which runs from "pressure" at the one end through "coercion" and ultimately to "force."

### WHEN EXPECTATIONS AND PRESSURE FAILED ...

For most of the men and women in our sample, the weight of expectation with some added pressure was "enough": enough to ensure that men got sex when their partners did not necessarily want it themselves; enough that on occasion men would accept refusals and resistance. In other cases, though, physical violence and/or threats were employed. Adele recalled how she was hit when she refused sex at her partner's mother's house, with her daughter downstairs. She describes how her partner was touching her leg and she said she didn't want to have sex with him after the abuse she had been experiencing. At first she felt trapped, knowing she did not want to, but simultaneously feeling as though she had to:

I thought 'Oh no, I don't want − don't want to', because that's how he made you feel. You'd think, 'You've put me through all this crap' ... all − all − physical and mental abuse, and now you want me to sleep with you! I'm thinking, 'No, no way!' But I've got to, or else he'd start again.

(Adele, Time 1)

On this occasion she decided she was going to make a stand, which prompted her partner to demand to know why she did not want to have sex with him. He told her to "fuck off downstairs," but put his foot in front of the door to prevent her from leaving. He then shut her arm in the door and she hit him in the eye. She instantly regretted it, as she knew it would result in more serious violence from him. "I'm thinking, 'Oh my God, what've I done?' And with that I just got boosh! round the face."

In some relationships physical assault and sexual violence were intertwined from the start. Holly recounted how her partner sat on top of her on the couch, holding her by her throat, trying to take her clothes off. On this occasion she tried to shout out for her daughter to come and help her, which she felt made him act even more brutally, and blamed her for their daughter potentially seeing him attempt to rape her.

> He said, "How dare you, you want [daughter] to see this?" and he put that all on me. Not considering the fact of what he was doing . . . "You're a fucking disgusting mother. You're shouting [daughter] you want [daughter] to see this?"
>
> (Holly, Time 1)

In Sophie's case no physical violence was ever used in the relationship, because her partner relied on coercive control. She discussed how, when they went on holiday, she would be plied with alcohol to dull her capacity for resistance. On one of these occasions she was so intoxicated that she did not realize until the day after what had happened when she ended up with a urinary infection. She challenged him over the phone when they got back.

> When we came home I said nothing and I actually challenged him on the phone 'cause I wouldn't do it to his face. I couldn't dare do it to his face, about taking advantage. And I did actually use the word rape and he called me sick. That was when a lot of the things came about. I said "Have you actually looked at the definition of rape? Even if someone's got consent through being drunk, drugs, or whatever, that is classed as rape and control." He lost the plot completely: "I'm sick? I'm getting the police onto you." He was getting the police onto me!
>
> (Sophie, Time 1)

Guy (Time 1) used coercive control (including emotional and verbal abuse and threats) in order to get what he wanted, including sex. He would also routinely threaten to make her homeless: "If you don't do this, I'll chuck you out of the house. If you don't do that, I'll chuck you out of the house." He acknowledged that he had used these threats to get anything and everything that he wanted: "all sorts – from sex, to ironing my clothes, to making my food."

Olive also talked about the impact of threats. On one occasion after her partner asked a seemingly innocuous question about a friend and Olive said she had heard from him earlier that day, she described how he "flipped," went "mental," and pinned her down on the bed.

> He said, "I'm going to fuck you up the arse and give you what you deserve." I was completely stunned and I think when it came out of his mouth I think it stunned him too because he immediately let me go. I went to get my bag and my things on the dressing table because I immediately wanted to leave. He stopped me from leaving. [Interviewer: How did he stop you from leaving?] He had hold of my arms and said "You are going nowhere, you are staying here."
>
> (Olive, Time 1)

### Sexual violence histories and herstories

In this section we describe two of the themes that were regularly brought up: participants' previous experiences of sexual violence, particularly as children, and the significance of pornography. As there were no specific questions about these issues, we cannot say how many of our participants had experienced previous sexual violence or used pornography, but these experiences formed an important context for those who did talk about these issues.

#### PREVIOUS EXPERIENCES OF SEXUAL VIOLENCE

Some of the men on the programs and the women partners and ex-partners described previous experiences of sexual violence when they were children. In addition, some of the women described sexual violence perpetrated by previous partners. Sometimes both partners in a relationship had experienced childhood sexual violence. Here we explore their reflections on the significance of these experiences within the current domestic violence context.

For the women, a common theme was having their experiences of sexual violence as children or in previous relationships used against them or integrated into the abuse perpetrated by their current partner or recent ex-partner. This was echoed by one of the men, Marlon, who recognized that he had used knowledge about his partner's previous domestic violence victimization, which included rape, to minimize his own behavior:

> From the beginning she used to turn around and say, "Why don't you just punch me instead of arguing with me and get it over and done with?" I then said, "You want me to punch ya, then carry ya up the stairs and have fucking sex with ya like ya ex used to?" I mean, he broke her ankle, he broke her arm, he threw her down the stairs, he broke her nose, you know, but she wouldn't have a bad word said against him.
>
> (Marlon, Time 1)

Some of the women interviewed had accessed specialist sexual violence services, often referred by their women's support workers (access to a women's support worker is a requirement of Respect-accredited perpetrator programs). It was in such contexts that they came to realize that their previous experiences played a part in their minimizing what was currently happening. "I've always, even from a small child, always been abused, very badly compared to – mostly physically and sexually, so [partner's] abuse didn't seem so dire" (Faye, Time 1).

Men tended to associated childhood sexual abuse (and in one case also sexual abuse as a young adult) with the way their sense of self had changed, often linked to misuse of alcohol, drugs, and engagement with pornography through teenage and early adulthood. Jeff explained how he used to be a selfish person, full of anger and hurt, who didn't give much thought to how his female partners were feeling.

> I think I had an issue with myself – hey, feeling vulnerable all the time, feeling like a victim, so when I was drinking I was sort of – that was emphasizing it and the underlying issues and it turned me into a nasty bugger myself. It gave me the confidence where I was not bothered about men, I'd inflict pain on anyone, do you know what I mean? . . . I had this thing in my head, "Do unto others what they have done to you," for years, and that's the way I sort of lived my life. But it's only my own time I've been wanting to be honest with you but it's a difficult thing to . . . it's not difficult to talk about it's just difficult to explain . . . where I have been at to where I am at now.
>
> (Jeff, Time 1)

Don revealed that both he and his partner had been sexually abused as children, but the impacts on them, in adult life, were very different.

> For me, sexually, it made me more aggressive, wanting more, chasing for more sexually, whereas my wife was the total opposite. My wife shut down. Her body shut down. So her mind, part of her mind, to do with sexuality also shut down.
>
> (Don, Time 1)

Although not all the participants identified the gender of the perpetrators who had sexually abused them previously, when it was identified it was always men. Hence, it may be important to recognize when working with men who use violence that a proportion will also have been harmed themselves by men's violence. It is also important for practitioners to bear in mind that some female partners will be dealing with previous experiences of domestic violence and childhood sexual abuse along with current abuse issues.

## THE SIGNIFICANCE OF PORNOGRAPHY

It was clear that pornography had been discussed within the DVPP group work. Some of the men talked about making jokes about pornography, but for many of them it was clear that this humor was masking something that they found it difficult to talk about within the group. Wayne, for example, talked about how he sometimes made light of the issue and joked with the group, but that he had also told the group outright that pornography was not a laughing manner and that he felt pornography was a problem for him.

> I access hard-core pornography because I hate myself. I have intensely, violently emotional swings and it hooks into it . . . I've still got the images in my mind when I'm with [partner]. Yeah, she's a willing participant, but where goes the gentle sex, where goes the loving sex, where goes that? That goes out the window.
>
> (Wayne, Time 2)

Men talked about how pornography had shaped their knowledge about sex and that this had led to them prioritizing their own needs over those of their partners. Don had recently made the decision to stop viewing any pornography as he now understood that what he had learned about sex through it had been damaging.

> I didn't have enough background . . . let's call it knowledge . . . on how to treat a woman, especially on the sexual side of it. You know, respecting her needs and wants, and I think really at that stage with this pornography giving you a false statement that the man goes in there . . . does his thing . . . and that's it. That is a totally wrong concept . . . totally, totally wrong. I've read quite a few books in the last couple of months and it has opened up my eyes to see what lies behind sexuality between couples . . . especially when couples love each other, not this pornography nonsense.
>
> (Don, Time 1)

Women at Time 1 referred to feeling it was impossible to live up to the standards that men expected through their viewing of pornography. Delia felt "detached" and "not involved" during sex, and unable to satisfy her partner sexually because she was not able to have what she called "porn star sex." Gwen was hurt that her partner was making comparisons with women in pornography: "When you see these women in the magazines they're not your typical woman you know they weren't like me; so I felt quite insignificant really."

Comments like these suggest that DVPPs and women's support workers need to factor the role of pornography in the work they do on sexual abuse and sexual respect and throughout other relevant parts of their interventions. See Chapter 13 for a more extensive discussion of the role of pornography in IPSV.

## Changes made/seen since attending the DVPP

We now highlight some examples where changes in relation to sexual respect were experienced by women or described by men. It seems that some modifications were starting to happen for those men who were using the program to *choose* to change their behaviors – although we are not suggesting that these changes were made by all the men.

It is relevant here to note that when asked in the Time 2 interviews which part of the program men found the most difficult, many named the sexual respect module. The content had made them particularly uncomfortable, and some did not see the point of it or consider it relevant to their behavior. Some did come to appreciate its relevance and importance, although a proportion of men continued at the Time 2 interview to distance themselves from sexually disrespectful behavior, associating it with "deviants" and claiming it had "nothing to do with me."

In the wider study, one of the changes that the programs made for some men was a much broader understanding of what constituted violence and abuse (Kelly & Westmarland, 2014), and the effects that more subtle, nonphysical forms of violence can have. This was also the case for sexual violence, with some men explaining that they now recognized behaviors, such as withholding affection, as forms of sexual abuse.

In the wider study we found that for men where the deepest changes in behavior toward their partner or ex-partner had been made, their way of relating to others such as friends, colleagues, and family also shifted. This was also the case for sexual respect, with Fred describing what took place when he was in a nightclub with a friend.

> He's there on the dance floor, grabbing girls' arses and all that, thinking it's highly hilarious and all that. And, you know, I just said to him, "Stop doing that because at the end of the day," I said, "They don't like it, and they don't want you grabbing their arses. If they – if they wanted you to grab their arse, they – they would've come up to you, or they would've made eye contact, they would have come and spoke to you or something like that." Obviously, you just don't go up to people grabbing their arses coz some people don't want it. Coz it's disrespecting them.
>
> (Fred, Time 2)

Similarly, Kieran described how he had come to understand what was meant by gender privilege and had started recognizing sexual disrespect in popular culture, giving examples such as topless models, pole dancing, and the book *Fifty Shades of Grey* as examples of sexual disrespect masquerading as female empowerment.

Some of the women also reported changes that they had experienced in relation to sexual respect. Delia, who had had significant problems with her partner coupled with past experiences of sexual violence, felt that a corner had been turned when interviewed at Time 2.

> Yes, what he has learnt is to respect it [sex]. He never respected it before. For him, it was like McDonald's, whereas in fact it's a three-course meal and he's had to learn the difference between the two. That sex in a marriage is not a McDonald's. It's a three-course meal.
>
> (Delia, Time 2)

Jill also described the sexual respect module as being a major turning point in the way her partner related to her.

> When he was doing the whole "Respecting Your Partner" and it came to obviously intimacy and that it opened his eyes and he came back and he was almost in tears and he was like, "Oh I'm sorry I have been like this with you. I can understand why you are the way you are" and all that. And I just sat there thinking, "Who are you and what have you done with [partner]?" sort of thing!
>
> (Jill, Time 2)

She went on to describe how he had originally denied that he had any problem with sexual respect and the way he treated her. This had completely changed. He now understood the need to take things slowly and be more patient, that his previous behavior continued to affect her.

While some men at the end of the program contended that the sexual respect module was of little relevance to them, others had absorbed the complex messages it contained and made significant adaptions both in their behavior toward their partner and in wider contexts.

## Conclusions

The purpose of this chapter was to start to shine a light on how sexual violence and sexual respect are dealt with within DVPPs in the UK. We attempted to review literature in the field as background information for this chapter and were surprised to find nothing similar existed. While some of our findings are tentative, and not as systematic as other parts of Project Mirabal, we offer this as a starting point for further research on the topic and as offering important themes for work with abusive men and their partners.

## References

Coy, M., Thiara, R., Kelly, L., & Phillips, R. (2011). Into the foreground: An evaluation of the Jacana Parenting Program. London CWASU. Retrieved from: www.niaending violence.org.uk/perch/resources/into-the-foreground-jacana-evaluation-report.pdf.

DVIP (2010). *Jacana parenting program manual*. Unpublished.

Kelly, L. (1987). *Surviving sexual violence*. Cambridge, MA: Polity Press.

Kelly, L., & Westmarland, N. (2014). *Domestic violence perpetrator programs: Steps towards change. Project Mirabal final report*. London and Durham, UK: London Metropolitan University and Durham University.

Philips, R., Kelly, L., & Westmarland, N. (2014). *Domestic violence perpetrator programs: An historical overview*. London and Durham, UK: London Metropolitan University and Durham University.

Stark, E. (2007). *Coercive control: How men entrap women in personal life*. New York, NY: Oxford University Press.

Westmarland, N., & Kelly, L. (2013). Why extending measurements of "success" in domestic violence perpetrator programs matters for social work. *British Journal of Social Wj203 ork*, *43*(6), 1092–1110.

Westmarland, N., Kelly, L., & Chalder-Mills, J. (2010). What counts as success? London, UK: Respect. Retrieved from: http://respect.uk.net/research/our-research-partnerships/mirabal-multi-site-evaluation-project.

# Chapter 19

# Law enforcement response to intimate partner sexual violence perpetrators

*Mike Davis*

## Introduction

With 24 years of experience in law enforcement, I have seen many changes in the way that intimate partner sexual violence (IPSV) is handled in the American criminal justice system. In this chapter, I share insights based on my experience dealing with IPSV perpetrators, including case examples. I explain how law enforcement can have an effective role with perpetrators while on scene at an IPSV crime, during the interview and follow-up, and when the perpetrator is in jail, in prison, or on probation or parole.

If there is one point to emphasize with any organization or jurisdiction for dealing with offenders, it is to have a coordinated community response that includes all relevant agencies and service providers. A coordinated community response comprises a team of individuals from various disciplines, agencies, and community partners who may have interaction with the IPSV victim, witnesses, and/or offender. A coordinated community response provides a well-informed, trained response to deal with IPSV in an effective way.

Everyone has a role to play in holding the perpetrator accountable. I have always felt that an abuser is relying on an uninformed community, inexperienced police officers on a busy shift who "buy" the perpetrator's story, a criminal justice system of prosecutors and courts that are not set up to deal with IPSV cases, victim advocates who may be uncomfortable with IPSV cases, and parole and probation officers who lack relevant training and work in isolation from the rest of the system. Myths about IPSV in general may also play a role. For example, IPSV is often viewed by the wider community, including some professionals, as being less serious than other forms of rape and sexual assault. These factors are what the offender is counting on. Don't be what the offender is counting on. There is too much at risk, including your own safety.

## Barriers for law enforcement

In the past, when intimate partner sexual abuse or sexual assault occurred in domestic violence cases, it was generally not asked about or dealt with. Most victims are uncomfortable talking about it and may feel humiliated. In many jurisdictions, law enforcement agencies, prosecutors, and courts have not been set up to receive the victim of IPSV so as to fully address this crime. Most perpetrators are counting on these factors to continue their crimes, and maintain power and control over the victim. As police officers and prosecutors try to better address the crimes of IPSV and domestic violence in the US, they have employed new strategies.

Law enforcement officers have seen a changing culture and awareness of IPSV cases. Many needed changes have come about. High-profile cases, legislative changes, police agency mandates, coordinated community response teams, and the impact of dangerous cases involving murder and suicide have heightened awareness of domestic violence that includes sexual assault. Professionals have begun to realize that if an abuser is threatening, hitting, or intimidating an intimate partner, sexual victimization is also likely. However, IPSV is so uncomfortable and horrific for most people to talk about that it has not been properly addressed. Many abusers know this.

Based on my experience, three major barriers to dealing with IPSV stand out. First, there was a lack of training for police officers on domestic violence and sexual assault in the past. When I was hired in 1991 and attended a big city police academy, we received very little training on domestic violence and sexual assault. I received virtually no training on IPSV, although I found that domestic violence calls were the most frequent violent crime I would go on during a patrol shift at a suburban police department. At the academy, we were given excellent training on the laws of arrest, search, and seizure, but at the time we simply did not know enough about IPSV and DV to properly train officers.

The second most significant barrier is the victim's difficulty in disclosing IPSV. Victims often are in fear, and may recant because of this (Bonomi, Gangamma, Locke, Katafiasz, & Martin, 2011). They think (with justification) that others will not look at IPSV as a crime. Describing demeaning sexual acts by their partner to others, especially the police and courts, may be incredibly difficult.

The third important barrier is that many jurisdictions (communities, police agencies, prosecuting attorneys) and courts are not set up to receive the victims when IPSV is reported or uncovered. The way the criminal justice system traditionally works can make it difficult to pursue these cases.

## Removing barriers and overcoming challenges

### A team approach

A significant change that has taken place to enhance the response of law enforcement, prosecuting attorneys, and communities to IPSV is the formation of specialized teams. Many of these teams are called Family Violence Justice Centers, or Family Justice Centers. According to the Family Justice Center Alliance (2016, para 1), these are:

. . . multi-agency collaboratives and multi-disciplinary models where victims of domestic violence, sexual assault, elder abuse, human trafficking, and other forms of violence can come [to] ONE PLACE. Family Justice Centers, and similar multi-agency, co-located service models, change the way the system works, simplifying and coordinating the web of service providers, so the system works more effectively for those in need.

In the jurisdiction where I work, the specialized unit is called the Domestic Violence Prosecution Center (DVPC). By collaborative agreement, police, prosecutors, victim advocates, parole/probation officers, child protection investigators, and other support staff use a team approach. At the DVPC in my jurisdiction we have an even more unique agreement in that our prosecutors, from both city and county agencies, are cross-deputized so that they can work felony *and* misdemeanor cases. This is significant in properly addressing IPSV. Many jurisdictions have different prosecutors for misdemeanor and felony cases. When IPSV is uncovered in what initially appeared to be a mis-demeanor (low-level) domestic violence case, a new prosecutor takes over when the newly discovered IPSV pushes the case to the level of a serious felony. In my jurisdiction, the case can be handled by the same prosecutor, without the complications of being revisited by different police, prosecutors, and advocates. In some cases, even the parole or probation officer may continue throughout the process after the offender's release from jail or prison.

Ultimately, this takes a real burden off the victim and holds the offender accountable because of the teamwork in a coordinated law enforcement and community response. This type of coordinated response has been identified as a best practice in response to both domestic violence and sexual assault (Clark, Lotz, & Alzuru, 2011). An extension of this unique approach is the formation of specialized domestic violence courts in which judges and support staff have training in domestic violence and IPSV.

### Asking about other crimes

Police now try to uncover all the circumstances and crimes that may be involved in a domestic violence case. One of these strategies is asking the victim about the totality and context of the crime or incident that brought her to the attention of the police. It also includes asking questions about other acts being committed against the victim and others, as well as the frequency and severity of those acts of abuse. This includes questions about forced sex or sexual assault. When we identify that forced sex did occur, we now incorporate a sexual assault investigation and protocol in our domestic violence investigation.

### Understand the victim, focus on the offender

As I have trained police officers, advocates, 911 dispatchers and other com-munity-based professionals about domestic violence in general and IPSV in particular, I emphasize that we have to understand why the victim is in fear and what that fear feels like to the victim. I train professionals not to get frustrated by the victim recanting or acting in ways we might not choose. Instead of focusing on "undesirable" victim response, we need to examine and focus on what the perpetrator does that causes the victim to recant or make choices that seem to be detrimental to the victim. Rather than ask, "Why does she stay?" we need to ask, "Why doesn't he stop abusing?" I focus on the offender's behaviors.

### Chronology of perpetrator contact

It is helpful to explore the steps in dealing with the perpetrator in chronological order, from the point where the IPSV case comes to the attention of the police and prosecutors, to its progress through the criminal justice system. Coercive and degrading sexual tactics are common in domestic violence cases whether there is overt IPSV or not (Logan, Cole, & Shannon, 2007).

### The initial contact

In most cases, someone calls police to report a domestic violence crime. Many times it is a witness, neighbor, passer-by, relative of the victim, or the victim. Police arrive on scene and begin an investigation. Police start asking questions to establish that a crime has been committed, evidence of the crime, witnesses to the crime, and information about the suspect or perpetrator.

In my experience it is very rare for a victim to call police and report being sexually assaulted by her intimate partner. It is so much easier for the victim to report a physical assault, telephone harassment, death threat, violation of a protection order, or damage to property than it is to report a sexual assault. There is much less humiliation with other crimes and the perpetrator is counting on that. Some victims do not know that IPSV is a crime because the perpetrator has told them that it is not a crime (National Center for Women & Policing, 2009). Another reason that a victim of IPSV may not know that a crime has occurred may be her own internalization of myths about IPSV, i.e, that "real" rape is when the perpetrator is a stranger.

### Uncovering other crimes

In many American jurisdictions, domestic violence victims are asked to complete a written statement. This statement asks questions about what was occurring, what has occurred in the past, and whether the victim is in pain, is fearful, or was injured. It also asks about threats, abuse of children, damage to property, abuse of animals, access to guns, past violence, and if the victim was forced to have sex. In my jurisdiction, the written statement not only asks about the crime, and the history and severity of the domestic violence, but also includes a series of questions in a "check the box" format asking if there has been forced sex.

This written statement offers the victim a less intimidating opportunity to disclose if sexual violence has occurred. Once we have a disclosure or evidence of IPSV, we as law enforcement can begin to deal with it. When police officers are unaware of all the crimes being committed upon the victim, the offender gets the cover they want, to avoid accountability. Many times there is a temptation for police, prosecutors, advocates, family members, and others to be satisfied with a simplistic domestic violence case and not explore the possibility of prior bad acts, especially something that is uncomfortable for many, such as sexual violence. An example of this: officers arrive on scene of a domestic violence call, learn that the victim was assaulted by being strangled by her boyfriend, and are satisfied with those facts alone. However, when we ask the right questions, we find the victim was also sexually assaulted just prior to the strangulation.

### Contacting the perpetrator on scene

Once the disclosure of sexual violence is received, police must begin addressing the sexual violence with the same tenacity as they would other felony crimes. If the perpetrator is on scene, steps should be taken so that the offender is sight and sound separate from the victim. It is a normal course of action for police to separate the victim and suspect. Police should begin documenting the condition of the suspect, just as they do the victim.

Officers should always read the victim statement on scene or as soon as possible to corroborate potential evidence and prepare for questioning of the suspect. On scene officers must find the right time at which the investigation turns from a reasonable suspicion that a crime has been committed to an arrest in which the suspect is in custody and not free to leave, and there is probable cause to place the suspect under arrest. This can move very fast on the scene of a domestic violence crime. Officers must administer the suspect their rights (the Miranda warning, in the US) when the suspect is in custody, or when the suspect would feel he is not free to leave and questions are asked of the suspect by police. Prepare to transport the suspect to a police station or jail where further interviewing, photos and suspect examination can take place.

### Preparing for the interview

Preparing to interview and question the suspect is done by documenting the excited utterances and/or spontaneous statements made by the suspect. Often these statements are made on scene, at the time of arrest, and during transport by police to a police station or jail. These statements are critical in countering potential defense claims made by the suspect. Officers should take photographs of the suspect and be prepared for a further examination of the suspect as details of the sexual violence emerge. Suspect examination has been lacking in many sexual assault cases in general and should be considered in IPSV cases, including forensic medical examination of the suspect if appropriate (Archambault, 2013).

In many cases of domestic violence, including IPSV, a thorough suspect interview is not conducted. Training in sexual assault investigation addresses the concern of suspect examination and varies depending on the jurisdiction. If there is an opportunity to record the interview with audio, or audio and visual records, this is preferred so that a transcript can be made of the interview and it can be used as evidence in the case.

There are many writings and trainings dedicated to interviewing. Rather than duplicate that work, I would like to point out a few tips specific to IPSV cases that had positive effects in cases I have encountered. First, I would interview many offenders on a weekly basis. These interviews were usually initiated soon after arrest. I was always eager to talk to the suspect to find out "why" and what happened. I had a sense of urgency to get the offender's story and statement before it all started to change. I wanted to know the truth about what happened, and see if the victim's safety and public safety were at risk for further violence. After many interviews over the course of more than six years, I came to some conclusions about effective preparation:

- Have a system set up to immediately interview the offender soon after arrest. I had computer alerts placed on suspects that I was looking for because I had probable cause to arrest, or they had arrest warrants issued for them.
- Get the interview done immediately. Upon police contacting the suspect, a specialized detective from the domestic violence unit or the case officer who is familiar with the case should be notified to initiate the interview.
- Prepare for the interview by reading the police reports, reviewing the photos and evidence, and having those items with you so you can confront the offender with them in the interview.
- Check the criminal history of the offender to get a better sense of their behavioral traits and dynamics of their behavior.

### Strategies for the IPSV perpetrator interview

An effective strategy is to have two officers present to interview. The secondary officer may be the offender's parole or probation officer. In my experience, this was always beneficial. The offender may respond to one officer better than another. A secondary officer may pick up on something missed by the primary interviewer. A parole or probation officer may be familiar with the suspect and have an understanding of the dynamics of the abusive relationship and any IPSV. A parole/probation officer can easily confront deception and may have a better observation on comparison and behavioral questions. I often ask the arresting officer to advise the suspect that a detective would like to talk with them to get their side of the story.

Usually, I introduce myself to the suspect, and express my concern and interest in the case and the suspect. I try to get the suspect some water and have him seated in a comfortable quiet place. Generally, this proves to be the interview room. There have been times when I have done a recorded interview with the suspect in the back of a police car, because at that moment the suspect wanted to talk and that was likely to change, so I seized the opportunity. Most interviews for IPSV cases are done in an interview room at the jail.

At the beginning of the interview I often ask questions that are nonadversarial so that I can get an observation of the suspect answering questions. I call these comparison questions. They provide the opportunity to observe the suspect's reaction and demeanor to questions that the offender can answer truthfully, then some that I know are not true. This is so that I can see what the offender is like when being deceptive.

In the interview, it is important to establish the dynamics of the relationship, such as where the couple met, if they have children in common, how long they have been together or lived together, who pays the rent, and who is vulnerable to abuse. I generally don't delve immediately into confrontational questions about the assault or sexual violence. I start by asking about the events of their day. After I let the suspect talk about this, I then confront with evidence, asking him why or how that could have happened.

### Considerations for interviewing the suspect

Based on my professional experience, I believe that being an abuser and batterer is a miserable life, which is why so many abusers threaten or commit suicide. It is not possible to truly control someone completely. An abuser cannot control a victim's thoughts or desires, which creates constant tension. When the victim separates from them or there is a chance of the abuser losing control, under circumstances such as arrest, divorce, child custody cases, or child protective services investigations, abusers resort to extreme and possibly fatal actions. Many times this includes suicide and taking someone with them – a partner, a child, a police officer, or someone else who has helped the victim.

### Three case examples

### Case 1

An adult female calls police to report being burglarized and assaulted by her ex-boyfriend, who is the father of her child. The ex-boyfriend is almost 17 years old. She reports that she had been out with her new boyfriend and returned home to find that her ex had broken into her apartment and was lying in wait for her to come home with the child they have in common. He then threatened her, assaulted her, cut her underwear off with a knife, and sexually assaulted her in front of their infant child.

The victim was taken to a hospital for exam. The apartment had broken glass where the suspect had cut himself and drips of blood were on the wall. The scene was not thoroughly examined by patrol officers. Detectives were called. The physical evidence at the scene and the collected evidence matched that of the victim's statement and witness statements.

The suspect had fled the scene but was located within a few hours of the sexual assault. He was visiting and staying with an acquaintance. The area where the suspect was found was searched for the knife. The suspect was placed under arrest and transported to a detention center for an interview by police. His clothing was taken as evidence, incident to arrest.

The interview with this 16-year-old suspect was lengthy and what appeared to be significant was the inability to contact any parent or guardian. One of his parents was deceased and the other was in prison. The suspect was very street smart and had been on his own for quite some time. He was living "under the radar," so to speak. He clearly understood his rights and wanted to speak with us.

He admitted the rape and violence after being confronted with the evidence. It was about halfway through the interview that this young man realized he was doing something wrong. He explained that his father was a violent abuser of his mother and used to hold a gun to her head in front of him. He equated relationships with violence.

This perpetrator received the counsel of a public defender. Consent was later given for DNA evidence to be taken from the suspect and he pleaded guilty to the IPSV. This case was an example of the need for a suspect exam to include photos, DNA swabs, and collection of clothing that could be tested for DNA. The interview was done with two officers; one officer was the original patrol officer called to the scene, and the other a detective in the domestic violence unit. The suspect made admissions when confronted with questions about specific sex acts after recounting the history of his background and the dynamics of his relationship with the mother of his child. This was a very disturbing and sad case, but it was dealt with in an effective manner.

## Case 2

In this case, a female was breaking up with her boyfriend. He assaulted her in a residence she shared with her parents. She was strangled by the suspect and then fled the residence and ran to a convenience store and asked the clerk for help and to use the phone. The abuser followed her into the store while she was on the phone with police. Police arrived and the abuser was arrested.

It was only after the victim started to complete the written domestic violence victim statement, administered by the responding officer, that the officer found out she had been raped as well as being strangled. The officer reviewed the statement on scene and immediately began a sexual assault protocol and investigation. The victim was transported to a hospital and domestic violence detectives were called.

The suspect was charged and pleaded guilty to a domestic violence crime. The victim did not want to pursue the rape charge. This case illustrates the need for first responders to ask the right questions and read the victim statement on scene. In this case the victim recanted, which is why it is so important to properly address all aspects of the crime. Identifying the sexual assault right away allowed the victim to receive proper medical attention and victim advocacy. Despite the eventual recantation, the complete investigation and sexual assault charges strengthened the case and plea agreement, leading to enhanced accountability for the perpetrator.

### Case 3

I recall a case that stands out because of the violence and the use of a defense commonly employed by perpetrators. A female victim ran to a neighbor's house, frantic, half-clothed, with her breasts exposed. She had been held against her will in the residence she shared with her boyfriend. He had terrorized her, punched holes in the walls, and set fires. Upon contact with the police he very confidently said, "She likes rough anal sex, with sex toys and strangulation." He then produced a collection of anal sex porn videos. In fact, the victim did engage in consensual rough sex in the past with him. Nonetheless, at this time the evidence was overwhelming that the victim was held against her will and terrorized in an act of physical and sexual abuse that was not consensual. The suspect had a criminal history that was unknown to the victim at the time. Detectives were called to the scene and the case was prosecuted by the specialized team, the Domestic Violence Prosecution Center.

From a police officer's perspective, this case highlighted an important point: many violent offenders find it so much easier to commit their violent acts on intimate partners. The intimate partner is often extremely vulnerable, fearful, and in the "clutches" of the abuser. Quite simply, why would a criminal take the risk of abusing a stranger when they believe it is easier to get away with hurting an intimate partner, because of so many barriers for the victim?

This case also demonstrates an important sexual assault investigation training point: a thorough and complete police investigation anticipates possible defense strategies and provides counters to them (Archambault, 2006). In cases of IPSV, the perpetrator's most common defenses may be that "she likes it rough," "she likes kinky sex," or that there is implied consent in the relationship. That is why it is so important to establish the dynamics of the relationship, who is vulnerable and why, along with the history and severity of any abuse and prior bad acts by the perpetrator. I always ask, "Who is scared of whom? And why?" Another significant strategy in dealing with perpetrators is listening to their jail phone calls (Bonomi et al., 2011). This can shed light on all these factors.

## Monitoring the perpetrator on parole or probation

Parole and probation officers are a part of the unique arrangement that is utilized in our specialized domestic violence unit at the Domestic Violence Prosecution Center. We had two probation officers assigned to the unit that worked cases with us, and we assisted them. These probation officers had a caseload of high-risk domestic violence offenders on parole and probation. The parole/probation officers assigned to the unit were experienced and received domestic violence training.

It was crucial to have officers assigned to the unit. A small percentage of criminals commit most crimes. Previous victims, the public, and potential future victims were in jeopardy if these high-risk offenders were not correctly monitored. Many of them violated protection orders, abused alcohol or drugs, and were arrested for violating the conditions of parole. It was common for police to arrive on scene and find that the suspect was on parole or probation. We could then notify one of these specialized officers and better address crimes such as IPSV.

I recall some of the most successful strategies we used. I had a partner in the unit who was a parole officer with a high-risk caseload. We would do a home visit of the offender on parole or probation; I would go for safety reasons. My partner was an experienced parole officer with extensive training in domestic violence. She would always make the offenders on her caseload disclose to their new spouse or girlfriend what they were on parole or probation for, making clear they were on probation for domestic violence crimes. We would meet with the new spouse or girlfriend and persons the offenders lived with, and respectfully ask questions in private about whether they were safe, at risk, or concerned about any abuse within the relationship. It would not be uncommon for us to uncover parole violations or find out about drug use, curfew violations, and new crimes. We would check on these offenders at off-hour times, when they would least expect us. Many times we would go in the evening, on a Sunday night, which was the most common time for domestic violence to occur. We would want to get a complete view of what was going on with a high-risk offender.

Our goal was victim safety, public safety, and officer safety. I have always felt that if a victim was not safe, then the public and police were not safe because of what that offender might do to the victim and others around them. We balanced our tactics. An example of this was my reaction to any parole violations of alcohol or drug use: I believed the offender should be immediately arrested. My partner's reaction was, "Let's arrest if it makes the victim, public, and police safer. If the offender loses his job because he is in custody over a minor violation, it may create more risk if he believes he has 'lost everything.'"

Most importantly, we communicated with the offenders' partners, and those victims who wanted to have a voice and be informed had a high level of confidence in us. We made many arrests to protect victims and we very rarely used force. I felt very confident that if a victim were being abused by an offender on parole or probation, they knew that they would be treated with respect if they confided in us, and some did. Although we had many cases that were resolved successfully, there were very violent habitual offenders who were serial abusers and went on to more victims. This demonstrates the dangerousness of IPSV offenders. For example, one offender raped his partner while she was pregnant. He was on probation for that and was later convicted of attempted murder in a nondomestic violence crime. He is now in prison.

## Conclusion

Law enforcement officers have a unique power that others in our society do not have – the power of arrest. That power of arrest includes bringing justice to the victims of a very challenging crime that has many barriers. In many cases, the police, prosecutors, and victim advocates are truly the ones pushing for this crime to be heard by a court, and advocating for safety in the victim's life and accountability for the offender.

## References

Archambault, J. (2006). Law and investigative strategy: What kind of sexual assault is this? Retrieved from the End Violence Against Women International website: www.evawintl. org/Library/DocumentLibraryHandler.ashx?id=39.

Archambault, J. (2013). Forensic exams for the sexual assault suspect. Training bulletin. Retrieved from the End Violence Against Women International website: www.evawintl.org/Library/DocumentLibraryHandler.ashx?id=2.

Bonomi, A.E., Gangamma, R., Locke, C.R., Katafiasz, H., & Martin, D. (2011). "Meet me at the hill where we used to park": Interpersonal processes associated with victim recantation. *Social Science & Medicine, 73*, 1054–1061.

Clark, M., Lotz, L.M., & Alzuru, C. (2011). *Best practices in the criminal justice response to domestic violence and sexual assault: Guidance for CCR/SART response protocols.* Durham, NC: North Carolina Coalition Against Domestic Violence and North Carolina Coalition Against Sexual Assault.

Family Justice Center Alliance. (2016). About the Family Justice Center Alliance. Retrieved from: www.familyjusticecenter.org.

Logan, T.K., Cole, J., & Shannon, L. (2007). A mixed-methods examination of sexual coercion and degradation among women in violent relationships who do and do not report forced sex. *Violence and Victims, 22*(1), 71–94.

National Center for Women & Policing (2009). Successfully investigating IPSV: Considerations for law enforcement. In Washington Coalition of Sexual Assault Programs (Ed.), *IPSV: Sexual assault in the context of domestic violence.* Olympia, WA: Washington Coalition of Sexual Assault Programs. Retrieved from: www.wcsap.org/sexual-assault-context-domestic-violence.

# Chapter 20

# Intimate partner sexual violence prevention with young people

*Kat Monusky and Jennifer Y. Levy-Peck*

## IPSV prevention: Too little, too late

Primary prevention of IPSV is a bold concept. Instead of prevention efforts aimed simply at identifying "warning signs" (Break the Cycle, 2014), primary prevention involves a complete reconceptualization of how to help young people have relationships free of intimate partner sexual violence, both in adolescence and throughout their lives. This includes but goes far beyond introducing ideas and skills related to healthy relationships. Using the socioecological model introduced below, prevention efforts need to target the underlying social beliefs and structures that serve as the soil in which sexually oppressive relationships grow.

Because intimate partner sexual violence (IPSV) occurs at the intersection of general intimate partner violence and sexual assault, it has not often been targeted for specific prevention efforts. In this chapter, we will consider evidence-based and promising approaches to sexual violence prevention, and discuss how they apply to the prevention of IPSV.

## What is prevention really?

Preventing sexual violence is a complex and nuanced component of the anti-sexual violence field. Prevention is an essential service, along with advocacy to survivors, long-term support, navigating medical and legal systems, policy reform, and other work as well. The label of prevention is often applied to a wide variety of activities and approaches, and is sometimes used interchangeably with education. However, many of the approaches labeled as prevention are better identified as raising awareness and risk reduction.

The public health model has become a valuable and widely used framework in sexual violence prevention work. By situating sexual violence prevention within this framework, we are able to draw on a model of identifying root causes and finding solutions to impact a large population of people, because the entire community is affected by sexual violence, regardless of direct survivorship (Centers for Disease Control and Prevention (CDC), 2004).

In order to create the largest impact, much of our work is focused on stopping the violence *before* it occurs. Public health work classifies prevention into three levels: primary (prior to sexual assault), secondary (immediate responses), and tertiary (long-term responses).

To meaningfully end the cycle of violence, we must develop efforts that are comprehensive and work on all the levels of prevention. Supporting survivors, reducing revictimization, and improving system responses are, of course, necessary components of creating social change. However, when most people think of the term *prevention,* what they are really hoping to achieve is primary prevention – preventing it from happening at all. This is why it is important that we accurately name the interventions we are using.

Primary prevention efforts address the root causes of sexual violence. In line with public health, this approach shifts the responsibility of prevention to society and away from victims (CDC, 2004). This approach requires us to look much deeper than the frequent superficial explanations that blame individual victims for the violence. Historically, and still today, we hear conversations and read media reports that attach sexual and intimate partner violence to the victim's clothing, alcohol or drug use, locality, reputation, and relationship status. However, primary prevention requires us to ask different questions about why violence happens.

## Getting to the roots

### Understanding perpetration to design prevention efforts

Without a framework to understand sexual violence, it can appear to be a crime that is hard to understand and potentially impossible to prevent. An important shift occurred in the anti-violence movement as researchers began to collect data to help dispel some of the myths about why sexual violence occurs. Extensive research with sex offenders/perpetrators has shown that, for the most part, sexual violence is not connected to individuals who are mentally ill, seeking sexual gratification, or unable to access sex (Scully, 1990). On the contrary, sexual violence is deeply entrenched in cultural acceptance and promotion of violence, commonly referred to as rape culture.

> What is rape culture? It is a complex of beliefs that encourages male sexual aggression and supports violence against women. It occurs in a society where violence is seen as sexy and sexuality as violent. In a rape culture women perceive a continuum of threatened violence that ranges from sexual remarks to sexual touching to rape itself. A rape culture condones physical and emotional terrorism against women as the norm. In a rape culture both men and women assume that sexual violence is a fact of life, inevitable as death or taxes. This violence, however, is neither biologically nor divinely

ordained. Much of what we accept as inevitable is in fact the expression of values and attitudes that can change.

(Buchwald, Fletcher, & Roth, 1993, p. xi)

Successful prevention efforts can develop within the shared understanding that sexual violence is deeply connected to a system of power and control (Lisak, 2011); therefore, these widespread norms and attitudes can be modified.

Primary prevention efforts focus on shifting key norms, attitudes, and beliefs of rape culture. National experts (Davis, Parks, & Cohen, 2006, p. 4) have focused on norms in five arenas that contribute to sexual violence:

- women (limited roles, objectification, and oppression);
- power (value on claiming and maintaining power, power over);
- violence (tolerance of aggression, victim blaming);
- masculinity (traditional constructs of manhood, domination, control and risk-taking); and
- privacy (the fostering of secrecy and silence).

These norms, while not exhaustive, help to illustrate the relationship between sexual violence and systems of oppression (Washington Coalition of Sexual Assault Programs & Guy, 2006).

### Gender issues: Yes, but . . .

Rape is inherently a highly gendered behaviour. The great majority of those who are sexually violent are men and the great majority of their victims are women. In the light of this, it is remarkable that gender as a notion is often not discussed in the empirical literature on perpetration. As a result, there has often been a failure to suggest that these attitudes may stem from a unifying underlying social ideology and value system, and equally a failure to posit that such a system may need to be changed if great strides are to be made in reducing rape perpetration.

(Jewkes, 2012, p. 23)

Jewkes's point is well taken: we must address the gender-based nature of intimate partner sexual violence if we wish to prevent it. All too often, however, this takes the form of thinking that we need only add prevention activities intended to stop male perpetration to the current array of activities aimed at preventing victimization for young women.

In fact, gender issues are far more complicated. Given the comparable rates of same-sex IPSV with IPSV in heterosexual relationships, the astronomical rates of sexual victimization of trans people, and the fact that people of all genders may subscribe to the "underlying sociology and value system" to which Jewkes refers (see, for example, Hird & Jackson, 2001), we must address these foundational issues rather than simply creating "his and hers" prevention curricula.

### Sexual entitlement and sexual obligation

The concept of sexual entitlement is a worldwide issue that underpins a great deal of sexual violence. (See also Chapter 5 for more discussion of entitlement and IPSV.) A 2013 United Nations study of 10,000 men in Asia and the Pacific found that

> The most common motivation that men cited for rape was related to sexual entitlement – a belief that men have a right to have sex with women regardless of consent. Men begin perpetrating violence at much younger ages than previously thought. Half of those who admitted to rape reported their first time was as a teenager.
>
> (UN Women, 2013, para 4)

In a study of adolescents in New Zealand, Hird and Jackson (2001) found:

> Male sexual need is understood to be so strong as to override what a girl-friend wants and leads to an interpretation of her protests as an impediment to be overcome. Such a construction of male sexuality excuses rape, attributing responsibility to biology rather than any "conscious" decision.
>
> (p. 36)

The IMAGES study, a five-nation research project addressing the factors that increase the likelihood of rape, found that men who had attitudes of sexual privilege and entitlement were more likely to rape, and also noted that men who perpetrated sexual violence were more likely to have been involved in a continuum of sexually aggressive behaviors as boys (Heilman, Hebert, & Paul-Gera, 2014).

In one of the few studies that explores teens' perceptions of the dynamic of sexual violence within intimate relationships, the researchers (in the UK) identified five common strategies whereby partners sexually coerced teen girls: "loss of partner, allusion to love, accusations of immaturity, manipulation of saying 'no' and fear tactics" (Barter, McCarry, Berridge, & Evans, 2009, p. 103).

Often, young people may be more concerned with pleasing or placating a partner than with identifying and meeting their own sexual desires. In a large-scale survey by Princeton Survey Research Associates International, 76% of teens who had oral sex said that the first time they did so, it was because their partner wanted to. A total of 22% of sexually active girls said their partner never performed oral sex on them, while only 5% of sexually active boys said so

(NBC News, 2005). This survey did not address any form of coercion other than "pressure."

Feeling pressure or obligation to have sex is not limited to females. A survey of black youth ages 13 to 21 showed that 54% of males stated they felt pressure to have sex (The National Campaign to Prevent Teen and Unplanned Pregnancy, 2011). The sense of obligation may come from a partner or from wider community expectations. Just as IPSV in marital or similar relationships may emanate from the belief that entering into a relationship is a "blank check" for sexual activity, sexual coercion in teen relationships may arise from beliefs on the part of either or both partners that, once in a relationship, the right to say "no" evaporates.

## Best practices for designing prevention approaches

We now turn to some guidance for the practical task of designing effective prevention programs. While the evidence for sexual violence prevention approaches is somewhat underdeveloped compared to other forms of public health prevention, there are best practice frameworks to rely on when designing approaches.

### The social ecological model

With the understanding that sexual violence is a complex problem and that it is woven into our social fabric, it only makes sense that our prevention strategies must be multifaceted and integrated into multiple personal and cultural spheres of life. That may sound like a daunting task, but with guidance from the public health framework called the social ecological model we have a roadmap to get started. The CDC utilizes a four-level model that consists of individual, relationship, community, and societal influences.

IPSV prevention is much more nuanced than other forms of public health problems, but the model is still applicable. When we use this model to understand IPSV for young people, we are able to see past the quick solutions that are sometimes appealing. We must focus on risk and protective factors at as many levels of the social ecology as we can in order to create the most potential for preventing IPSV. For example, we might design a program to teach empathy skills and explore the continuum of gender expression and norms with young people while also building a community of gender equity through policy, media, and engagement activities.

### Risk and protective factors

Drawing on research from the public health field helps in designing programs that reduce risk factors and promote protective factors for perpetration. These risk and protective factors are not causal, but contributing; they do not guarantee an individual will or will not perpetrate violence. These factors are useful, however, in selecting key messages or approaches that may lessen the likelihood of violence. While some of the identified risk factors, such as poverty or prior victimization or perpetration are not easily modifiable by prevention programming, others can help direct programming focus areas.

The CDC (2015) routinely conducts research and analyzes data about risk and protective factors for sexual violence. The following selection of risk factors for sexual violence perpetration may be especially relevant to intimate partner sexual violence in the lives of young people, as many can be modified or influenced during adolescence.

- **Individual risk factors:** Alcohol and drug use; delinquency; empathetic deficits; acceptance of violence; early sexual initiation; exposure to sexually explicit media; hostility toward women; adherence to traditional gender role norms; and hyper-masculinity.
- **Relationship factors:** Emotionally unsupportive family environment; poor parent–child relationships; association with sexually aggressive, hyper-masculine, and delinquent peers; involvement in a violent intimate relationship.
- **Community factors:** Lack of support from police and judicial system; general tolerance of sexual violence within the community; weak community sanctions against sexual violence perpetrators.
- **Societal factors:** Norms that support sexual violence; norms that support male superiority and sexual entitlement; norms that support women's sexual submissiveness; weak policies related to gender equity.

The current literature on protective factors for sexual violence is not as robust as the research on risk factors; however, these factors can still be useful in designing programming. The CDC (2015) includes the following: parental use of reasoning to resolve conflict; emotional health and connectedness; academic achievement; and empathy and concern for how one's actions affect others.

### The nine principles

One of the most widely accepted measures for designing effective prevention programs comes out of research from Nation et al. (2003). While this research was not exclusively about gender-based forms of violence, the findings have been widely adopted within our field. These principles prescribe the structure and delivery methods of prevention programming, not the content. It may feel overwhelming to meet these standards, but they serve as a useful checklist (summarized from Nation et al., 2003):

1. **Comprehensive services** (multiple components and settings, range of protective factors).

2.  **Varied teaching methods** (include active, skills-based component).
3.  **Sufficient dosage** (enough exposure to have an effect).
4.  **Theory driven.**
5.  **Positive relationships** (foster strong, stable, positive relationships between children and adults).
6.  **Appropriately timed** (for maximum developmental impact).
7.  **Socioculturally relevant** (tailored to cultural beliefs and practices, community norms).
8.  **Outcome evaluation.**
9.  **Well-trained staff.**

## What is not working in prevention

### The "dating violence" label

Much of the violence prevention work being done with young people in the United States and elsewhere is framed as the prevention of "dating violence." The coining of that term has been helpful in that it has expanded the concept of domestic violence to include unmarried partners, but it often does not resonate with young people, nor does it bring to mind the continuum of sexual violence within relationships that we seek to prevent.

Teen relationships are varied and changing. The traditional notion of a "date" – in which a well-dressed boy shows up at a girl's home, meets her parents, is instructed to have her home by midnight, treats her to a movie, perhaps engages in some limited form of physical affection, and then asks her out for a specific time in the future – bears little resemblance to the lives of most young people today.

In addition, the use of the word "violence," while often defined to include sexual aggression, does not immediately bring to mind sexual coercion or assault. Like the term "domestic violence," "dating violence" is often considered to consist of physical assault. The more subtle forms of intimate partner sexual violence, such as sexual coercion or pregnancy pressure (see Chapter 11), certainly don't fit into common notions of dating violence.

### Raising awareness or reducing risk as prevention

It can be challenging to understand the different types of outreach programming: awareness, risk reduction, and primary prevention. The two key elements that set these series of approaches apart are the intended goal or outcome and the level of dosage (Washington Coalition of Sexual Assault Programs, 2015).

Historically communities have been resistant to addressing sexual and intimate partner violence, but more recently they have begun to welcome some level of education for young people especially. Unfortunately, the type of programming often requested, such as assemblies or information sessions, has not been found to be effective as prevention. One-hour and one-time programs are not effective at preventing perpetration: "None of these have shown lasting effects on sexual violence risk factors or behavior" (National Sexual Violence Resource Center, 2014, p. 3).

**Awareness programs and events** seek to raise community understanding, and hopefully lower acceptance, of sexual violence. For example, a school-based awareness program about teen IPSV might be a series of classroom sessions that provide an overview and definitions of teen dating violence, discusses "red flags" of unhealthy or unsafe relationships, and identifies what help is out there for those experiencing this violence. These programs are a wonderful first step for a community to break silence and secrecy about existing violence and improve system response to holding perpetrators accountable. These are often (but not always) one-time events.

**Risk reduction** seeks to lower an individual's vulnerability by having them look for signs of potential violence, and change their behavior. For example, a risk-reduction approach to teen sexual assault might be a weekend workshop hosted in the community or at a local school teaching young women basic self-defense skills and practicing assertive techniques to say "no."

These programs may be effective to prevent some individual experiences of sexual violence, but they do not target the source of the problem (the perpetrator) and therefore will not have community-wide impact. This approach may convey the message to potential victims, largely girls and women, that sexual violence is unavoidable and their responsibility, which may lead to internal and community-wide victim blaming. Risk reduction programs often omit sexual violence that takes place in the context of an ongoing relationship and is part of a wider pattern of coercive control (Morrison, Hardison, Mathew, & O'Neil, 2014).

All these programs and activities can be valuable for young people; however, they have been found ineffective in creating the level of change needed to prevent sexual violence (CDC, 2016). Anti-violence organizations are typically doing a great deal of work with only a limited amount of resources. Therefore, it is important to identify and plan activities correctly to get to the desired outcomes.

### Sweeping it under the rug

Ignoring sexual violence sends a dangerous message. The current focus on campus sexual violence has highlighted the lax enforcement of sanctions for sexual assault. University officials have often dismissed sexual misconduct claims, particularly in the context of an ongoing relationship, with the attitude that "boys will be boys," or the idea that somehow rape is simply the result of miscommunication (Charleswell, 2014; Krakauer, 2015). In middle and high schools, despite the current focus on bullying prevention, school administrators often overlook sexual harassment and sexual violence as an important segment of bullying experiences (Jones, 2015).

## Prevention that works

As mentioned above, one of the most recent and robust studies about the effectiveness of sexual violence prevention strategies is a 2014 report from the CDC. The researchers examined 140 primary prevention studies between 1985 and 2012 that met the level of rigor to be included (DeGue et al., 2014). From this large pool of studies, only two programs were identified as showing effective results in reducing sexually violent behavior for young people: *Safe Dates* and *Shifting Boundaries*.

> Safe Dates (Foshee and Langwick, 2010) is a dating violence prevention program for middle- and high school students. It includes a 10-session curriculum, a play, and a poster contest. Students were significantly less likely to self-report sexual violence victimization or perpetration in dating contexts four years after participating in the program.
>
> (NSVRC, 2014, p. 3)

*Shifting Boundaries* (National Institute of Justice, n.d.) building-level intervention is part of a dating violence prevention program for middle schools that involves environmental changes, a poster campaign, "hotspot" mapping, and school staff monitoring. There is also a classroom curriculum. The building-level intervention (but not the curriculum) reduced self-reported perpetration and victimization of sexual harassment and sexual violence among peers, and decreased self-reported sexual violence victimization" (NSVRC, 2014, p. 4).

As the *Shifting Boundaries* program (discussed in detail in Chapter 21) demonstrates, appropriate institutional response is an important component of creating a safer environment for young people (primary prevention) and reducing rates of sexual harassment and assault (secondary and tertiary prevention).

It is important to note that these pre-made programs are unlikely to work for all communities, so prevention staff should review the programs to determine if they are a good fit (NSVRC, 2014). In fact, the principles of effective prevention require tailoring curricula to their intended audiences (DeGue et al., 2014). Even though there is limited evidence of what is working to prevent sexual violence, adhering to the best practices for designing prevention programs is an important step to build the evidence base we need.

## Our vision

### Prevention begins in infancy

Jewkes (2012, p. 3) states that "some risk factors for raping start from birth," and it is therefore essential to "strengthen care giver child attachment, reduce use of physical punishment, and enhance parenting."

Heilman, Hebert, & Paul-Gera (2014) concur:

> Many of the most consistent influences on men's likelihood of perpetrating sexual violence occur during childhood and adolescence. Policies and programs aiming to prevent violence must therefore place greater emphasis on setting a nonviolent life course among young children and adolescents.
> (p. 14)

Ensuring a healthy environment for every child, free from child abuse and witnessing other family violence, is a critical component of prevention (Kahn & Paluzzi, 2006).

Obviously, prevention efforts directed at very young children do not directly target sexual behavior. Instead, we need to direct our attention to developing the characteristics that would make sexual perpetration unlikely throughout the lifespan, particularly with a relationship partner:

- Secure attachment and ability to form healthy emotional bonds.
- Healthy relationship boundaries (both sexual and nonsexual).
- Respect for others.
- Ability to take responsibility for one's actions.
- Self-respect.
- Humility (as opposed to an attitude of entitlement).
- Acceptance and valuing of diversity.
- Flexible approach to gender roles and expectations.
- Capacity for empathy.
- Self-control and the ability to delay gratification.
- Age-appropriate knowledge about relationships and sex.
- Ability to follow reasonable rules and laws.
- Emotional self-regulation.

These characteristics are consistent with CDC protective factors (2015) that prioritize nonviolent conflict resolution and respectful, caring interactions with others. It is hard to imagine a young person who possesses most or all of these characteristics engaging in sexual violence. Taking responsibility for one's actions may be a particularly salient factor. In a survey of adolescents, two-thirds of those who admitted perpetrating sexual violence stated that it was entirely or partially the victim's fault (Ybarra & Mitchell, 2013). This study (in which 75% of the victims were romantic partners) also showed that perpetration of sexual violence begins early, with an upswing in perpetration at age 16. Those who perpetrated were more likely to have been exposed to explicit sexual media and somewhat more likely to have been exposed to violent but nonsexual media. A primary lesson here is that what happens to children early in life is critical in preventing sexual violence in adolescence and adulthood.

## Putting it all together

Here is what we know: Sexual violence prevention efforts must begin early; must address individual, relationship, community, and societal factors; must be consistent with the principles of effective prevention set forth by the CDC; and must clearly target IPSV along with other forms of sexual abuse and assault. By now, we should have moved far beyond "prevention" programs that warn of "stranger danger," tell girls and young women to protect themselves, and fail to address the underlying societal factors that increase the risk of perpetration.

## References

Barter, C., McCarry, M., Berridge, D., & Evans, K. (2009). Partner exploitation and violence in teenage intimate relationships. Retrieved from the National Society for the Prevention of Cruelty to Children website: www.nspcc.org.uk/globalassets/documents/research-reports/partner-exploitation-violence-teenage-intimate-relationships-report.pdf.

Break the Cycle (2014). Warning signs. Retrieved from: www.breakthecycle.org/warning-signs.

Buchwald, E., Fletcher, P., & Roth, M. (1993). Preamble. In E. Buchwald, P. Fletcher, & M. Roth (Eds.), *Transforming a rape culture*. Minneapolis, MN: Milkweed.

Centers for Disease Control and Prevention (CDC) (2004). *Sexual violence prevention: Beginning the dialogue*. Atlanta, GA: Centers for Disease Control and Prevention.

Centers for Disease Control and Prevention (CDC) (2015). Sexual violence: Risk and protective factors. Retrieved from: www.cdc.gov/violenceprevention/sexualviolence/riskprotectivefactors.html.

Centers for Disease Control and Prevention (CDC) (2016). Sexual violence: Prevention strategies. Retrieved from: www.cdc.gov/violenceprevention/sexualviolence/prevention.html.

Charleswell, C. (2014, July 2). Boys will be boys: America's campus rape policy. The Hampton Institute. Retrieved from: www.hamptoninstitution.org/americas-campus-rape-policy.html.#V_4RPY-cGUK.

Davis, R., Parks, L.F., & Cohen, L. (2006). Sexual violence and the spectrum of prevention: Towards a community solution. Retrieved from the National Sexual Violence Resource Center website: www.nsvrc.org/publications/nsvrc-publications/sexual-violence-and-spectrum-prevention-towards-community-solution.

DeGue, S., Valle, L.A., Holt, M.K., Massetti, G.M., Matjasko, J.L., & Tharp, A.T. (2014). A systematic review of primary prevention strategies for sexual violence prevention. *Aggression and Violent Behavior*, 19, 346–362.

Foshee, V., & Langwick, S. (2010). *Safe dates: An adolescent dating abuse prevention curriculum* (2nd ed.). Center City, MI: Hazelden.

Heilman, B., Hebert, L., & Paul-Gera, N. (2014). *The making of sexual violence: How does a boy grow up to commit rape? Evidence from five IMAGES countries*. Washington, DC: International Center for Research on Women (ICRW) and Promundo.

Hird, M., & Jackson, S. (2001). Where "angels" and "wusses" fear to tread: Sexual coercion in adolescent dating relationships. *Journal of Sociology*, 37, 27–43.

Jewkes, R. (2012) *Rape perpetration: A review*. Pretoria: Sexual Violence Research Initiative. Retrieved from the Sexual Violence Research Initiative website: www.svri.org/Rape Perpetration.pdf.

Jones, L.M. (2015, August). Violence prevention and school climate program implementation in the school district of Philadephia. In K.M. Edwards & L.M. Orchowski (Co-chairs), *Theoretically driven approaches to reducing interpersonal violence among youth and young adults.* Symposium conducted at the meeting of the American Psychological Association, Toronto, Canada.

Kahn, A., & Paluzzi, P. (2006). Boys will be boys: Understanding the impact of child maltreatment and family violence on the sexual, reproductive, and parenting behaviors of young men. Washington, DC: Healthy Teen Network. Retrieved from: www.healthy teennetwork.org/sites/default/files/Boys_Will_Be_Boys.pdf.

Krakauer, J. (2015). *Missoula: Rape and the justice system in a college town.* New York, NY: Doubleday.

Lisak, D. (2011). Understanding the predatory nature of sexual violence. *Sexual Assault Report, 14*(4), 49–57.

Morrison, S., Hardison, J., Mathew, A., & O'Neil, J. (2004). *An evidence-based review of sexual assault preventive intervention programs.* Research Triangle Park, NC: RTI International. Retrieved from: www.ncjrs.gov/pdffiles1/nij/grants/207262.pdf.

Nation, M., Crusto, C., Wandersman, A., Kumpfer, K.L., Seybolt, D., Morrissey-Kane, E., & Davino, K. (2003). What works in prevention: Principles of effective prevention programs. *American Psychologist, 58*, 449–456.

The National Campaign to Prevent Teen and Unplanned Pregnancy (2011). Almost half of black youth report pressure to have sex: New ESSENCE magazine/national campaign survey released. Retrieved from: http://thenationalcampaign.org/press-release/almost-half-black-youth-report-pressure-have-sex.

National Institute of Justice (n.d.). Program profile: Shifting Boundaries. Retrieved from Crime Solutions: www.crimesolutions.gov/ProgramDetails.aspx?ID=226.

National Sexual Violence Resource Center (2014). Key findings from "A systematic review of primary prevention strategies for sexual violence perpetration." Retrieved from: www.nsvrc.org/publications/nsvrc-publications-guides-research-briefs/key-findings-systematic-review-primary.

NBC News (2005). Nearly 3 in 10 young teens "sexually active." Retrieved from the NBC News website: www.nbcnews.com/id/6839072#V_457o-cGUK..

Scully, D. (1990). *Understanding sexual violence: A study of convicted rapists.* New York, NY: Harper Collins Academic.

UN Women (2013). UN survey of 10,000 men in Asia and the Pacific reveals why some men use violence against women and girls. Retrieved from UN Women website: http://asiapacific.unwomen.org/en/news-and-events/stories/2013/9/un-survey-of-10000-men-in-asia-and-the-pacific.

Washington Coalition of Sexual Assault Programs (2015). Moving further upstream. Retrieved from: www.wcsap.org/moving-further-upstream.

Washington Coalition of Sexual Assault Programs, & Guy, L. (2006). Rape culture. *Partners in Social Change, 9*(1). Retrieved from: www.wcsap.org/rape-culture.

Ybarra, M.L., & Mitchell, K.J. (2013). Prevalence rates of male and female sexual violence perpetrators in a national sample of adolescents. *JAMA Pediatr., 167*(12), 1125–1134. doi:10.1001/jamapediatrics.2013.2629.

# Chapter 21

# Preventing sexual violence and sexual harassment with young people

## A one-year follow-up on the *Shifting Boundaries* intervention

Bruce G. Taylor, Elizabeth A. Mumford,
Weiwei Liu, and Nan D. Stein

## Introduction

Rigorous data has emerged documenting the effectiveness of primary prevention programs in middle schools to reduce adolescent sexual violence.[1] However, questions still remain on the "dosage level," or number of sessions, that must be sustained for these programs for adolescents, such as one semester of interventions in a single year or two dosages across two years, to produce violence reductions. Also, it is unclear if schools could implement these types of programs in just one grade (as opposed to multiple grades in middle schools) to conserve resources but still achieve the violence reduction effects. This chapter describes a study done in New York City schools, building on previous research with a program called *Shifting Boundaries,* which has been demonstrated to be effective in reducing teen sexual dating violence and harassment. This study addresses how often to intervene, and how broadly to intervene across grade levels in middle schools (grades 6, 7, and 8) in order to reduce sexual violence and sexual harassment.

## Prior research

Increasingly, teen sexual dating violence and sexual harassment (SDV/H) have been viewed as significant problems in the violence prevention fields (Centers for Disease Control and Prevention, 2014; Schubert, 2015; Taylor & Mumford, 2014 e-pub ahead of print). Terminology varies when considering these issues. We use the term *dating violence and harassment* (DV/H) to represent physical, emotional, or sexual abuse within a dating relationship, the definition that CDC used for teen dating violence (Centers for Disease Control and Prevention, 2014). Where cited studies used the term *teen dating violence,* we also follow the language of the original research. See Chapter 20 for a discussion of terminology regarding adolescent sexual violence. We will also use the term

DV/H to also cover youth sexual harassment, as defined by the American Association of University Women (Hill & Kearl, 2011).

Local and regional studies reveal that approximately 50–60% of teens are victims of teen dating violence (Foshee, 1996; Hickman, Jaycox, & Aranoff, 2004; Jouriles, Platt, & McDonald, 2009; Malik, Sorenson, & Aneshensel, 1997; O'Keefe, 1997). As of 2014, drawing on the national Survey of Teen Relationships and Intimate Violence (STRiV), one in five reported physical and/or sexual victimization, while one in eight adolescents reported perpe- trating physical and/or sexual violence in a dating relationship (Taylor & Mumford, 2014 e-pub ahead of print). In addition to the risk of physical injury, teen dating violence is associated with significantly poorer mental and physical health (Howard, Wang, & Yan, 2007) and is a risk factor for adult intimate partner violence (Berkowitz, 2010; Gomez, 2010).

Among adolescents, along with increases in dating behavior, the onset of puberty is accompanied by increases in sexual harassment (Pepler et al., 2006), which may occur within or outside dating or peer relationships. The 2011 AAUW study found in a nationally representative sample of youth (12–18 years old) that about half of their sample reported being a past-year victim of sexual harassment (Hill & Kearl, 2011).

### Interventions

A number of interventions have been developed to prevent teen dating violence (TDV) and rigorous research has been conducted on their effectiveness (Foshee & Reyes, 2009; Jaycox et al., 2006a; Taylor et al., 2010a; Wolfe et al., 2009). However, most of the rigorous studies on these interventions have been undertaken in North America, and the extent to which these programs are transferable to other settings and cultures is uncertain (Stanley, Ellis, Farrelly, Hollinghurst, & Downe, 2015). Also, these studies are few and generally address only students who are about 13 or 14 years old or older (Foshee et al., 1998; Jaycox et al., 2006b; Wolfe et al., 2009). Only a few addressed 6th and 7th grade students, who are typically about 11 or 12 years old (Peskin et al., 2014; Taylor et al., 2010a). Only two other TDV experiments, outside the *Shifting Boundaries* experiments (Taylor, Stein, & Burden, 2010a, b; Taylor, Stein, Mumford, & Woods, 2013) have been done exclusively with middle school students (Cissner & Ayoub, 2014; Peskin et al., 2014). Also, *Shifting Boundaries* is the only one of these interventions that is also designed to prevent adolescent sexual harassment.

A curriculum called *Safe Dates* has experimentally shown a reduction in long- term physical dating violence (Foshee et al., 2005). In another of the more rigorously evaluated interventions (the *Fourth R*), Wolfe and colleagues (2009) found that after 21 sessions, the program for the 9th grade Canadian students was able to reduce physical dating violence in the intervention group as compared to the control group up to 2.5 years post-treatment. In a randomized controlled trial evaluation with ten middle schools in southeast Texas (n = 766 students), Peskin and colleagues found that those receiving the TDV prevention program called *It's Your Game . . . Keep It Real* (IYG) experienced less physical TDV victimization and emotional TDV victimization, and perpetrated less emotional TDV than the control group (Peskin et al., 2014). In another randomized controlled trial evaluation of the *Fourth R* with ten Bronx, NY middle schools (Cissner & Ayoub, 2014), the study showed *no impact* of the *Fourth R* on dating violence, peer violence/bullying, or sexual violence (Cissner & Ayoub, 2014).

### Shifting boundaries experiments

The study we report on in this chapter builds on two earlier experiments of the *Shifting Boundaries* (SB) intervention. In 2005, our team conducted one of the first experimental evaluations of a primary prevention program addressing sexual dating violence and harassment for 6th- and 7th-grade students in suburban middle schools bordering Cleveland, Ohio. The research team randomly assigned 123 study classrooms to one of three conditions:

- Treatment 1, an interaction-based curriculum that addressed SDV/H by focusing on setting and communicating boundaries in relationships, the formation of respectful and mutual relationships/friendships, and the role of the bystander as intervener.
- Treatment 2, a law and justice curriculum that addressed SDV/H by focusing on laws, definitions, information, and data about penalties for sexual assault and sexual harassment, as well as results from research about the consequences for perpetrators of gender violence.
- Control group that went through the normal class schedule and did not receive any of the elements of treatment 1 or treatment 2.

This earlier research in Cleveland confirmed that SDV/H reductions could be achieved with middle-school prevention programming (Taylor, Stein, Mack, Horwood, & Burden, 2008; Taylor et al., 2010a).

From 2008 to 2010, in New York City (NYC) middle schools, the team conducted a second experiment (Taylor, Stein, Mumford, & Woods, 2013). In this study ("NYC-1"), our team added a building-wide intervention component (labelled *Shifting Boundaries* Schoolwide, or SBS) to go along with the most effective components of the Cleveland classroom-based interventions. Our team randomly assigned 30 public middle schools to one of four conditions: (1) receive the SBS and *Shifting Boundaries* classroom (SBC) interventions; (2) receive SBS only; (3) receive SBC only; or (4) control group (no interventions). The main findings from this study were that the building-only and the "both" (classroom lessons with building-wide) interventions were effective at reducing sexual dating and peer sexual violence victimization and perpetration (Taylor et al., 2013).

A couple of key questions remained from the NYC-1 experiment: first, whether the SB program was of sufficient dosage to produce sustained effects after the intervention, beyond the six months demonstrated in NYC-1; and second, if schools could implement the SB program in just one grade to conserve resources but still achieve SDV/H reduction effects. While the Safe Dates evaluation (Foshee et al., 2004) had assessed the question of dosage (and found no additional TDV reductions associated with a booster session), we did not find another study in the literature that explored the effects of providing an intervention across the middle school grades versus one grade receiving a SDV/H intervention.

In 2011, the same team started a third experiment (the "NYC-2" study). The NYC-2 study extended the earlier work in Cleveland and NYC-1 by:

- expanding the study to include 8th grade as well as 6th and 7th grade students;
- including the use of a few lessons from Safe Dates (Foshee et al., 1998) for 8th grader students;
- testing revised grade-specific DV/H interventions for middle schools (our earlier work used classroom lessons that were not specific to a certain grade level);
- and having a longer follow-up period of 12 months instead of the six months follow-up of the NYC-1 research.

This chapter describes the one-year follow-up results using sexual violence/harassment outcome measures.

## How the study was conducted

We randomly assigned 23 public middle schools in NYC to one of four SB treatment conditions. Unfortunately, only 13 of these 23 schools (and 814 students) were able to continue in our study for the one-year follow-up period, yielding a similar sample size as the Foshee *Safe Dates* experiment which had 14 schools (Foshee et al., 1998). The unit of assignment and unit of analysis were schools – in other words, the schools themselves were considered the subjects in this study, along with the individual students.

We examined schools which received varying levels of dosages of SB (inclusive of SBC and SBS interventions):

- **Group 1:** Schools assigned here received SB in one school year for 6th graders only.
- **Group 2:** Schools received SB in one school year for their 6th and 7th grades.

- **Group 3:** Schools received SB in one school year for their 6th, 7th and 8th grades.
- **Group 4:** Schools received SB over two school years first in 6th grade and the same group received it in 7th grade the following school year.

The classroom intervention was delivered through a multi-session curriculum that emphasized the consequences for perpetrators of DV/H, state laws and penalties for DV/H, and respectful relationships. The school (building-level) based intervention included the development and use of temporary school-based restraining orders (respecting boundaries agreements), higher levels of faculty and security presence in areas identified by students and school personnel as unsafe "hot spots," and the use of posters to increase awareness and reporting of DV/H to school personnel.

We had to modify our planned design for this experiment due to low levels of participation among the NYC middle schools. While we planned to have a no-treatment control group, it proved not to be feasible. We decided to maximize our use of the schools to address our main research question of the comparative effectiveness of different levels of SB treatment. Also, we had a no-treatment control group with our NYC-1 experiment conducted only a couple of years before the current study and it had already addressed the effectiveness of the intervention (treatment versus no-treatment[2]).

We had hoped to have our 6th-grade longitudinal group receive three years of treatment. However, too few of the schools were willing to continue participation beyond two years of treatment due to competing academic demands within the schools and staffing deficits leading to a resistance to applying limited resources to DV/H prevention. Similarly, we had hoped to have up to a 24-month follow-up survey, but that plan had to be abandoned given the lack of willingness of schools to continue participation. The schools agreed to a one-year of follow-up surveys. Nevertheless, the one-year follow-up was a longer follow-up period than the earlier research on SB that only had a six-month follow-up period (Taylor et al., 2008; Taylor et al., 2013; Taylor et al., 2010a). Despite these modifications in the original design, we believe some important findings emerged from this study.

### Description of participants

Participants ranged in age from 10 to 15, with a nearly 50% split between boys and girls. Our sample was 27% Hispanic, 36% African American, 15% Asian, 15% White and 7% "other." Over 40% of the sample had prior experience with a violence prevention educational program. Nearly half reported at least one experience of being in a dating relationship. At baseline, about one in five respondents reported having ever been the victim of any physical dating violence, with a similar number reporting perpetrating any physical dating violence. One in ten respondents reported having been the victim of any sexual dating violence ever (about 6.5% for perpetration of this act). Almost 60% of the sample reported having ever been the victim of any physical peer violence at some point in time (45% perpetration), and 18% were ever the victim of sexual peer violence (8% perpetration). Also, 49% reported experiencing SH at some point in time (23% perpetration).

We had three schools and 128 students in Group 1 (6th grade only), two schools and 227 students in Group 2 (6th and 7th grades), four schools and 225 students in Group 3 (6th, 7th and 8th grades) and four schools and 234 students in Group 4 (two years of treatment).

## Measures

### Sexual harassment

SH is defined as unwanted sexual behavior portrayed as comments, images, or gestures that are sexual in nature. The term includes comments or behavior regarding someone's gender identity in terms of sexual preference or physical development (Hill & Kearl, 2011). The surveys measured prevalence of the experience of being a victim and/or perpetrator of SH.

### Sexual violence

While SH also includes extreme behavior such as rape (Hill & Kearl, 2011), school-based prevention research has often measured sexual violence on distinct scales. Measures of peer violence, both in terms of victimization and perpetration (Taylor, Mumford, Liu, & Stein, 2015), are based on surveys developed specifically for assessing the impact of sexual violence prevention programs (Foshee et al., 1998; Schewe, 2000; Ward, 2002). Our survey included prevalence (yes/no) and frequency questions (e.g., *How many times did you do this to them in the past 6 months? Zero times? 1 to 3 times? 4 to 9 times? 10 or more times?*). The questions covered the experience of being a victim and/or perpetrator of sexual violence by/of peers and a separate set of questions about dating partners. Because of sensitivity concerns raised by school personnel regarding explicit measurement of sexual violence in a middle-school population, we were limited to two main *sexual violence* items ("pushed, grabbed, shoved, or kicked you in your private parts" and "made you touch their private parts or touched yours when you did not want them to"), similar to other research (Foshee et al., 1998). The survey also included a small number of background variables about the students, including age, gender, and ethnicity/racial background and questions on prior attendance at an educational program about sexual assault, harassment, or violence, and prior history of dating.

We were able to successfully show the effects of our interventions through our data analysis by ensuring that our treatment groups were comparable at the outset of the study and that we had the minimum number of required participants to make reliable and valid comparisons (Taylor et al., 2015). We also made adjustments in our statistical models to allow for the clustered nature of our data (i.e., we have students who share some similar background characteristics by virtue of attending the same school and living in similar social environments).

For the most part, the four study groups/conditions were similar on the majority of our measures, leaving the only major differences across the groups their assigned condition (Taylor et al., 2015). Additionally, random assignment procedures were followed closely. All schools assigned to treatment received their appropriate treatment. We used statistical methods to address any pre-treatment differences. While there was attrition in our study, it did not create any observable patterns of bias that interfered with our ability to draw inferences from the results (Taylor et al., 2015).

### Study structure

We examined whether more exposure to the SB program led to greater reductions in SDV/H than a single intervention and looked at the effects of presenting the program in more than one grade versus a single grade only. We looked at the 12-month follow-up information. For these analyses we have three groups:

- **a 6th-grade only group** (n = 3 schools with 128 students) which serves as our reference group in our models;
- **a 6th-grade longitudinal group** (n = 4 schools with 234 students), that received the 6th-grade intervention when they were in 6th-grade and the 7th-grade intervention when they were in 7th grade;
- **a multi-grade group:** schools assigned to receive the 6th- and 7th-grade SB intervention (n= 2 schools) or the 6th, 7th and 8th grade (n = 4 schools) SB intervention (combined n = 6 schools and 452 students for both sets of schools).

The current study builds on two prior studies of the *Shifting Boundaries* program, one of which was conducted in the same study population of NYC middle schools. In our prior multi-level research of the *Shifting Boundaries* program (NYC-1) – classroom curricula (SBC) and building-wide activities (SBS) – we found that the building-wide and the combined building-wide and classroom curricula interventions were effective at reducing SDV/H victimization and perpetration (Taylor et al., 2013).

### Results

Our NYC-2 results indicate that, overall, providing the SB treatment to only one grade level in a middle school generally does just as well in terms of peer sexual violence and dating sexual violence outcomes as a more saturated process of treating multiple grades in the school.

There were no results indicating that offering the SB program to a grade of students in two successive years (the 6th-grade longitudinal design) resulted in *statistically* differential effects compared to a one-time delivery of the program in 6th grade. This finding is analogous to Foshee and colleagues' study that found no additional TDV reductions associated with a booster session delivered two years (our intervention was one year later) after the original application of the intervention (Foshee et al., 2004). While Foshee and colleagues (2004) did not find any additional benefits of an extra dosage, additional booster effects have been detected with other adolescent problem behavior interventions related to smoking prevention (Botvin, Renick, & Baker, 1983; Dijkstra, Mesters, De Vries, Van Breukelen, & Parcel, 1999) and substance use (Botvin, Baker, Filazzola, & Botvin, 1990; Spoth, Redmond, & Shin, 2001).

At the 12-month assessment, however, there was evidence that additional saturation beyond one grade is associated with reductions in SH victimization. Schools that delivered SB to 6th, 7th and 8th graders or both 6th and 7th graders (compared to just 6th graders) showed reductions in SH victimization reports at 12 months. However, we also found that greater saturation of the SB program (delivered to 6th and 7th graders or to all three grades levels) was unexpectedly associated with *more* reported perpetration of sexual violence against peers at 12-month post treatment compared to the 6th grade only group. This higher level of reporting of perpetrating sexual violence against peers could mean that the program itself increased this form of violence. It is also possible that we might have a reporting effect issue. That is, the intervention sensitized students to recognizing when they were perpetrators of sexual violence, so they were more likely to report this on the survey. Under this interpretation, the intervention is helping students recognize these acts as violence and perhaps increasing the sensitivity of this group of participants to the illicit nature of sexual violence and improving their likelihood of reporting this form of violence.

Another alternative, the most likely case, is that it could be a spurious finding because it is not supported by other examples of increases in violent behavior associated with greater saturation of SB. In fact, this finding stands in contrast with the additional borderline statistically significant findings ($p < .10$) that delivering the program to 6th graders in year 1 and again to the same students, as 7th graders, in year 2 was associated with less SH victimization frequency compared to the 6th grade only intervention. This highlights the potential value of multiple dosages of the SB program for SH prevention work. Nevertheless, in sum, the weight of evidence suggests that increased SB program dosage over the middle school years is not indicated to address peer and dating sexual violence and SH outcomes.

Our full results are available in our project final report (Taylor et al., 2015).

## Limitations

The general limitations of self-reports are applicable to this study such as recall issues with the timing of a violent act or deliberate under-reporting of certain insidious behavior (Jackson, Cram, & Seymour, 2000), or over-reporting/ exaggerations of certain behavior. Next, because of concerns raised by school personnel on the sensitivity of such questions for a middle-school population, we were limited in how we could measure sexual victimization to two main items. Also, our study was limited at the upper end to a 12-month follow-up period, and it is unclear whether our findings would change over a longer follow-up period.

Another major concern in our study was whether attrition in our study created any pattern of bias that would interfere with our ability to draw unequivocal inferences from our study. Overall, we did not observe much by way of patterns in our study for the schools that continued on to complete the follow-up survey waves and those schools that dropped out after doing only a baseline survey. As reported in our final report (Taylor et al., 2015), we observed few differences between the dropout schools and the completer schools on a variety of background factors and violence measures. Where there were some differences, we addressed this in our statistical modeling.

## Implications and conclusion

Despite the difficulties of completing the NYC-2 study, and the associated changes we had to make to the study, we still believe some important new knowledge emerged. We learned after NYC-2 that for the most part, delivering the program more frequently and over a longer period of time does not alter the findings for our SDV/H outcome measures compared to just implementing the SB program with 6th-grade students only. Our results largely support a minimalistic approach, in that SB effectiveness may be achieved by delivery to only one grade level in middle schools. Providing the SB treatment once in 6th grade works as well as applying it once per year for two years with the same group (in 6th and 7th grades). Likewise, implementing SB with only one grade level in a middle school does just as well in terms of SDV/H outcomes as a more saturated process of treating multiple grades in the school.

However, we did find that additional saturation beyond one grade is associated with reductions in SH victimization at the 12-month follow-up period. Considering our NYC-1 and NYC-2 results together, we believe there is empirical justification for a saturated implementation of the school-wide component SBS across the entire school environment. That is, we feel the data support implementing the SB program for at least the 6th-grade students; given the nature of the SBS building intervention, that aspect can be extended to the whole school with little extra cost.

What remains to be examined in the future are protocols to support school maintenance of SBS activities beyond the research phase, and the development of ongoing assessment and administrative efficiency measures. Also, while SB is a full program to prevent SDV/H in school settings, it would still need to be adapted and aligned with local conditions, just as we did first in Cleveland and later in New York City. Just as for other off-the-shelf youth violence prevention programs that can be very influential (Stanley et al., 2015), a strong argument can be made for using SB as a starting point for a community to begin to combat youth SDV/H. SB provides a framework and could be integrated into other ongoing local efforts to combat youth SDV/H. Our team worked with youth, teachers and administrators in developing SB. Similarly, these same types of stakeholders could be presented with SB and given an opportunity to have their voices integrated into a locally adapted version of SB, with co-produced materials.

As outlined in the Stanley review (Stanley et al., 2015), we also found that organizational readiness is key to implementing SDV/H interventions. SB is a straightforward program to implement but, in our assessment, only if a school is ready to embrace change in the school environment and not accept SDV/H as an inevitable feature of the experience of adolescence. Adolescence is a critical developmental juncture and SB offers an opportunity to proactively address the problem of intimate partner violence, including sexual violence, through primary prevention before it becomes deep-rooted and becomes a destructive part of adulthood.

## Acknowledgments

The study on which this chapter is based ("A dating violence prevention program for each grade in middle school: A longitudinal multi-level experiment") was funded by the National Institute of Justice (NIJ) (Grant 2010-MU-MU-0008). The views expressed are those of the authors and do not necessarily represent the views or the official position of NIJ or any other organization.

We are grateful for the funding of the NIJ and how it allowed us to continue our testing of the *Shifting Boundaries* program. We thank our Project Officer Dr. Carrie Mulford and Senior Grants Management Specialist Laurie Bright for their encouragement and support. We would like to express our gratitude to the principals, staff, and students at all our participating schools, for this research would not have been possible without their help. Thanks also to those at the NYC Department of Education who helped to make this research possible. In particular, Scott Bloom, LCSW (Director of School Mental Health Services, Office of School Health, NYC Department of Education) was instrumental with helping our team locate schools interested in participating in this research. We would like to acknowledge the rest of the *Shifting Boundaries* team, including Keith Towery for all his work on managing the project logistics.

## Notes

1. In the U.S., the term "middle school" refers to educational institutions for students approximately ages 10–13; they generally encompass either two or three grade levels prior to secondary education.
2. The authors use "treatment" here to refer to the SB interventions, not therapeutic treatment.

## References

Berkowitz, A.D. (2010). Fostering healthy norms to prevent violence and abuse: The social norms approach. In K.L. Kaufman (Ed.) *The prevention of sexual violence: A practitioner's sourcebook* (pp. 147–171). Holyoke, MA: NEARI Press.

Botvin, G.J., Baker, E., Filazzola, A D., & Botvin, E.M. (1990). A cognitive-behavioral approach to substance abuse prevention: One-year follow-up. *Addictive Behaviors, 15*(1), 47–63.

Centers for Disease Control and Prevention (2014, March 19). Understanding teen dating violence fact sheet. Retrieved from: www.cdc.gov/violenceprevention/pdf/teen-dating-violence-2014-a.pdf.

Cissner, A.B., & Ayoub, L.H. (2014). Building healthy teen relationships: An evaluation of the Fourth R Curriculum with middle school students in the Bronx. U.S. Department of Justice.

Dijkstra, M., Mesters, I., De Vries, H., Van Breukelen, G., & Parcel, G. (1999). Effectiveness of a social influence approach and boosters to smoking prevention. *Health Education Research, 14*(6), 791–802.

Foshee, V.A. (1996). Gender differences in adolescent dating abuse prevalence, types and injuries. *Health Education Research, 11*(3), 275–286.

Foshee, V.A., & Reyes, H.L.M. (2009). Primary prevention of adolescent dating abuse: When to begin, whom to target, and how to do it. In J. Lutzker & D. Whitaker (Eds.), *Preventing partner violence* (pp. 141–168). Washington, DC: American Psychological Association.

Foshee, V.A., Bauman, K.E., Arriaga, X.B., Helms, R.W., Koch, G.G., & Linder, G.F. (1998). An evaluation of Safe Dates, an adolescent dating violence prevention program. *American Journal of Public Health, 88*(1), 45–50.

Foshee, V.A., Bauman, K.E., Ennett, S.T., Linder, F., Benefield, T., & Suchindran, C. (2004). Assessing the long-term effects of the safe dates program and a booster in preventing and reducing adolescent dating violence victimization and perpetration. *American Journal of Public Health, 94*(4), 619–624.

Foshee, V.A., Bauman, K.E., Ennett, S.T., Suchindran, C., Benefield, T., & Linder, G.F. (2005). Assessing the effects of the dating violence prevention program "Safe dates" using random coefficient regression modeling. *Prevention Science, 6*(3), 245–258.

Gomez, A.M. (2010). Testing the cycle of violence hypothesis: Child abuse and adolescent dating violence as predictors of intimate partner violence in young adulthood. *Youth & Society, 43*(1), 171–192. doi: 10.1177/0044118x09358313.

Hickman, L.J., Jaycox, L.H., & Aranoff, J. (2004). Dating violence among adolescents: Prevalence, gender distribution, and prevention program effectiveness. *Trauma, Violence, and Abuse, 5*, 123–142.

Hill, C., & Kearl, H. (2011). *Crossing the line: Sexual harassment in schools.* Washington, DC: AAUW.

Howard, D.E., Wang, M.Q., & Yan, F. (2007). Psychosocial factors associated with reports of physical dating violence among US adolescent females. *Adolescence*, 42(166), 311–324.

Jackson, S.M., Cram, F., & Seymour, F. (2000). Violence and sexual coercion in high school students' dating relationships. *Journal of Family Violence*, 15(1), 23–36.

Jaycox, L.H., McCaffrey, D., Eiseman, B., Aronoff, J., Shelley, G.A., Collins, R.L., & Marshall, G.N. (2006a). Impact of a school-based dating violence prevention program among Latino teens: Randomized controlled effectiveness trial. *Journal of Adolescent Health*, 39(5), 694–704.

Jaycox, L.J., McCaffrey, D.F., Ocampo, B.W., Shelley, G.A., Blake, S.M., Peterson, D.J, Richmond, L.S., Kub, J.E. (2006b). Challenges in the evaluation and implementation of school-based prevention and intervention programs on sensitive topics. *American Journal of Evaluation*, 27(3), 320–336.

Jouriles, E.N., Platt, C., & McDonald, R. (2009). Violence in adolescent dating relationships. *The Prevention Researcher*, 16, 3–7.

Jouriles, E.N., Mueller, V., Rosenfield, D., McDonald, R., & Dodson, M.C. (2012). Teens' experiences of harsh parenting and exposure to severe intimate partner violence: Adding insult to injury in predicting teen dating violence. *Psychology of Violence*, 2(2), 125.

Malik, S., Sorenson, S.B., & Aneshensel, C.S. (1997). Community and dating violence among adolescents: Perpetration and victimization. *Journal of Adolescent Health*, 21(5), 291–302.

O'Keefe, M. (1997). Predictors of dating violence among high school students. *Journal of Interpersonal Violence*, 12, 546–568.

Pepler, D.J., Craig, W.M., Connolly, J.A., Yuile, A., McMaster, L., & Jiang, D. (2006). A developmental perspective on bullying. *Aggressive Behavior*, 32(4), 376–384. doi: 10.1002/ab.20136

Peskin, M.F., Markham, C.M., Shegog, R., Baumler, E.R., Addy, R.C., & Tortolero, S.R. (2014). Effects of the It's Your Game . . . Keep It Real Program on dating violence in ethnic-minority middle school youths: A group randomized trial. *American Journal of Public Health*, 104(8), 1471–1477. doi: 10.2105/AJPH.2014.301902.

Schewe, P.A. (2000). Report of results of the STAR project to the Illinois Violence Prevention Authority. Chicago, IL.

Schubert, K. (2015). Building a culture of health: Promoting healthy relationships and reducing teen dating violence. *Journal of Adolescent Health*, 56(2), S3–S4.

Spoth, R.L., Redmond, C., & Shin, C. (2001). Randomized trial of brief family interventions for general populations: Adolescent substance use outcomes 4 years following baseline. *Journal of Consulting and Clinical Psychology*, 69(4), 627.

Stanley, N., Ellis, J., Farrelly, N., Hollinghurst, S., & Downe, S. (2015). Preventing domestic abuse for children and young people: A review of school-based interventions. *Children and Youth Services Review*, 59, 120–131.

Taylor, B., & Mumford, E.A. (2014 e-pub ahead of print). A national descriptive portrait of adolescent relationship abuse: Results from the National Survey on Teen Relationships and Intimate Violence (STRiV). *Journal of Interpersonal Violence*, 1–26. doi: 10.1177/0886260514564070.

Taylor, B., Stein, N., Mack, A.R., Horwood, T.J., & Burden, F. (2008). Experimental evaluation of gender violence/harassment prevention programs in middle schools. Washington, DC: National Institute of Justice.

Taylor, B., Stein, N., & Burden, F. (2010a). The effects of gender violence/harrassment prevention programming in middle schools: A randomized experimental evaluation. *Violence and Victims*, 25, 202–223.

Taylor, B.G., Stein, N., & Burden, F. (2010b). Exploring gender differences in dating violence/harassment prevention programming in middle schools: Results from a randomized experiment. *Journal of Experimental Criminology*, 6(4), 419–445. doi: 10.1007/s11292-010-9103-7.

Taylor, B., Stein, N., Mumford, E., & Woods, D. (2013). Shifting boundaries: An experimental evaluation of a dating violence prevention program in middle schools. *Prevention Science*, 14(1), 64–76. doi: 10.1007/s11121-012-0293-2.

Taylor, B., Mumford, E., Liu, W., & Stein, N. (2015). Assessing different levels and dosages of the Shifting Boundaries intervention to prevent youth dating violence in New York City middle schools: A randomized control trial. Washington, DC: National Institute of Justice.

Ward, K.J. (2002). Making the invisible visible: A feminist evaluation of an adolescent gender violence prevention program. Doctoral dissertation. Cornell University. Ithaca, NY.

Wolfe, D.A., Crooks, C., Jaffe, P., Chiodo, D., Hughes, R., Ellis, W., Stitt, L. and Donner, A. (2009). A school-based program to prevent adolescent dating violence: A cluster randomized trial. *Archives of Pediatrics & Adolescent Medicine*, 163(8), 692–699. doi: 10.1001/archpediatrics.2009.69.

# Chapter 22

# Conclusion

## A fresh approach to prevention, identification, and accountability of intimate partner sexual violence perpetrators

*Jennifer Y. Levy-Peck, Patricia Easteal, and Louise McOrmond-Plummer*

> A problem inadequately named cannot be adequately addressed.
> (Carol J. Adams, *I just raped my wife!*
> *What are you going to do about it, Pastor?*)

We raise our daughters to look for rapists in parking lots, in dark alleys, and in crowded bars. Seldom do we tell them: look in the movie seat next to you where your boyfriend holds your hand; look across the altar to the man who is saying his wedding vows to you; look at the father of your newborn baby, smiling in your hospital room. And yet, these may be the rapists who will damage their lives. These may be the rapists who are held in high esteem in the community, who tell people their partners are crazy, who are given a wink and a nod as they describe forced sex, who seldom spend a night in jail, and who generally fly under the radar of our social institutions.

Who are these men and why did we write a book about them? The answer is simple: communities, governments, and programs will not end victimization by focusing only on survivors. Perpetrators commit the acts, and learning about perpetration is the only path to effective prevention and intervention. When we ignore those who perpetrate intimate partner sexual violence (IPSV), we ignore our best chance for preventing a huge proportion of sexual assaults. We miss the chance to identify a significant risk of death to women who are in relationships with physically violent men who also sexually harm them. We also ignore the pain and distress of children who are exposed to a toxic atmosphere of sexual oppression as they grow up. And, while we focus solely on their victims/survivors, partner rapists evade accountability for their crimes.

In considering perpetrators, it is wise to avoid "either/or" thinking: either they are monsters, or they are damaged human beings; either they are individually responsible, or this is a social problem; either practitioners provide treatment, or they engage the criminal justice system; either the focus is on addressing the underlying factors that fuel perpetration, or on educating our communities about safety.

The range of contributions in this book point to an alternative lens – instead of the "either/or" perspective, we see from a holistic and flexible perspective the value of a "both/and" view. These perpetrators commit monstrous acts, and they are indeed human beings; learning about their motivations and psychological characteristics does not mean that we excuse their behavior. We can look at the social context of IPSV while holding perpetrators personally accountable. We can research effective interventions, often in the context of treatment mandated by the courts. We can and must provide community education, while also working to eliminate the societal factors that fuel gender-based violence in general, and IPSV in particular.

The basic concepts for addressing IPSV, as outlined below, are distilled from the experts who have contributed to this book. Each chapter adds to the picture of what constitutes IPSV and what we can do about it.

## Step one: Shifting our focus

> As one of the primary needs of victims is for their sense of justice and fairness to be restored in so far as possible, holding the perpetrator to account is a core aspect of serving the victim. It also serves the needs of society and ultimately the long-term good of the perpetrator.
>
> (Ireland's *Second National Strategy on Domestic, Sexual and Gender-Based Violence*)

The focus must shift to perpetrators and their impact. Survivors are often a "convenience sample" for researchers. Only a tiny fraction of IPSV offenders enter the criminal justice system or seek treatment on their own. Researchers and practitioners need to develop innovative ways to reach men and boys in the general population who believe that they "own" the women and girls in their lives and have carte blanche to force, coerce, or manipulate them into unwanted sexual activity.

This does not mean, of course, that the needs of survivors and their children should be overlooked. Robust efforts to help with healing and recovery are critical, and resources should not be diverted from programs to support survivors. Yet in many cases, the reality is that the perpetrators will remain in the lives of these survivors and children, or will move on to other relationships with the potential for victimization; therefore, including perpetrators in our efforts to create change is vital.

## Step two: Learning to recognize IPSV in all its forms

> In order to escape accountability for his crimes, the perpetrator does everything in his power to promote forgetting. If secrecy fails, the perpetrator

attacks the credibility of his victim. If he cannot silence her absolutely, he tries to make sure no one listens.

(Judith Lewis Herman, *Trauma and Recovery*)

The next step is to clearly recognize and identify what constitutes IPSV and what strategies abusers may use, as we have done in several chapters of this book. Their tactics may range from emotional pressure to engendering fear of death. For decades, people have been asking domestic violence survivors "Why do you stay?" Similarly, there is a lack of understanding (by both community members and professionals) of the dynamics of IPSV and the reasons why an adult would remain in a relationship with a sexual abuser. The harrowing survivor stories in this volume are there for a reason: they illuminate the many ways in which sexual violence is manifested in intimate partnerships.

IPSV can take place both in the context of a physically violent relationship, and also as a stand-alone form of abuse. This knowledge is important because remedies that address only those perpetrators who are also batterers will miss those who use other forms of coercion, manipulation, and force.

### Step three: Looking at the big picture

Rape culture is a complex set of beliefs that encourage male sexual aggression and supports violence against women.

(Emilie Buchwald, *Transforming a Rape Culture*)

A number of contributors have provided examples of how perpetrators are condoned by individuals and institutions. From peer support for "scoring" sexually to indifference from the courts, perpetrators and potential perpetrators get the message that it is no big deal to sexually abuse a partner.

A particularly disturbing trend is the upsurge in violent, misogynistic pornography that normalizes sexual violence and teaches young people a callous disregard for emotional connection and mutual respect in sexual relationships. In the absence of comprehensive sex education, this is how many adolescents learn about sexuality and intimate relationships.

We cannot single out perpetrators for study and intervention without looking at the cultures in which they live. IPSV is a worldwide problem that is rooted in oppressive attitudes and institutionalized gender bias.

### Step four: Requiring accountability

Requiring accountability while also extending your compassion is not the easiest course of action, but it is the most humane, and, ultimately, the safest for the community.

(Brené Brown, *Rising Strong*)

Effective interventions must be identified and developed. These men live in our communities. Very few of them will spend any significant amount of time in prison. They may still be loved by their partners and their families. They are fathers and brothers and sons as well as husbands and boyfriends.

Innovative curricula for batterer intervention programs are a promising start. Because of the prevalence of sexual assault by domestic violence perpetrators, all batterer intervention programs should include a focus on sexual respect and consent, along with the more broad-based learning about gender-based violence. In addition, sexual offender treatment programs should evaluate and address sexual violence against partners, past or present, regardless of whether IPSV was the proximate cause for entering treatment. Since most perpetrators who receive treatment do so because they are court-ordered, judges and community corrections officers need to know about appropriate interventions for IPSV, along with mental health professionals and substance abuse treatment providers. IPSV perpetrators have specialized treatment needs, and more research needs to be conducted to determine the most effective interventions.

Accountability also means better training for law enforcement, to ensure thorough investigation of possible IPSV and a prepared response when sexual assault is disclosed. Multidisciplinary community teams that include law enforcement, advocates, and prosecutors minimize trauma to victims, and make prosecution more likely. Both criminal and family court personnel must also receive adequate training so that perpetrators can be held accountable and their partners and children can be protected.

## Step five: preventing IPSV through community action

> Human nature is complex. Even if we do have inclinations toward violence, we also have inclination to empathy, to cooperation, to self-control.
>
> (Steven Pinker)

We need to raise our children in an atmosphere of respect and safety. The messages young people get throughout childhood and adolescence are relevant to reducing the risk of perpetration and victimization. Accurate and age-appropriate information about sexuality, reduction and effective treatment of trauma to children, measures to promote gender equality, clear expectations of respectful behavior, and reasonable consequences for any form of sexual aggression are common-sense methods for reducing the prevalence of IPSV.

Religious congregations and schools are among the community institutions that can stand strong against IPSV by making it clear that this behavior is not to be tolerated and by connecting individuals with community resources. They can provide broad-based education about equality and consent, along with sanctions for those who jeopardize individual and community safety through sexual violence.

It is our hope that the perspectives, information, and insights provided by this book will assist readers, no matter what their professional or community role, in taking the necessary steps forward to reduce the perpetration of intimate partner sexual violence.

Each of us should be safe in our own homes, in our own beds, and in the lives we share with our partners. It is up to everyone, from parents of young children to judges in all nations' highest courts, to work toward the elimination of intimate partner sexual violence.

# Index

Please note that italics denote figures; bold denotes boxes

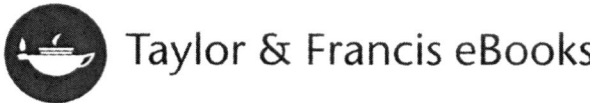

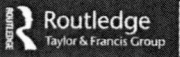